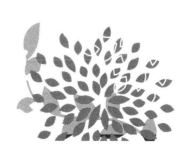

BLOOM

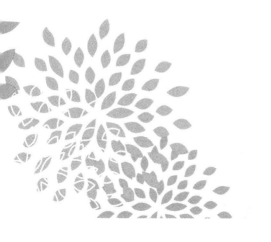

ALSO BY BRONNIE WARE

The Top Five Regrets of the Dying

Your Year for Change

All of the above are available at your local bookstore,
or may be ordered by visiting:

Hay House UK: www.hayhouse.co.uk
Hay House USA: www.hayhouse.com®
Hay House Australia: www.hayhouse.com.au
Hay House South Africa: www.hayhouse.co.za
Hay House India: www.hayhouse.co.in

BLOOM

A Tale of Courage, Surrender and Breaking Through Upper Limits

Bronnie Ware

HAY HOUSE

Carlsbad, California • New York City • London
Sydney •Johannesburg • Vancouver • New Delhi

First published and distributed in the United Kingdom by:
Hay House UK Ltd, Astley House, 33 Notting Hill Gate, London W11 3JQ
Tel: +44 (0)20 3675 2450; Fax: +44 (0)20 3675 2451; www.hayhouse.co.uk

Published and distributed in the United States of America by:
Hay House Inc., PO Box 5100, Carlsbad, CA 92018-5100
Tel: (1) 760 431 7695 or (800) 654 5126
Fax: (1) 760 431 6948 or (800) 650 5115; www.hayhouse.com

Published and distributed in Australia by:
Hay House Australia Ltd, 18/36 Ralph St, Alexandria NSW 2015
Tel: (61) 2 9669 4299; Fax: (61) 2 9669 4144; www.hayhouse.com.au

Published and distributed in the Republic of South Africa by:
Hay House SA (Pty) Ltd, PO Box 990, Witkoppen 2068
info@hayhouse.co.za; www.hayhouse.co.za

Published and distributed in India by:
Hay House Publishers India, Muskaan Complex, Plot No.3, B-2,
Vasant Kunj, New Delhi 110 070
Tel: (91) 11 4176 1620; Fax: (91) 11 4176 1630; www.hayhouse.co.in

Distributed in Canada by:
Raincoast Books, 2440 Viking Way, Richmond, B.C. V6V 1N2
Tel: (1) 604 448 7100; Fax: (1) 604 270 7161; www.raincoast.com

A catalogue record for this book is available from the British Library.

ISBN: 978-1-78180-732-3

Printed and bound in Great Britain by CPI Group (UK) Ltd, Croydon CR0 4YY

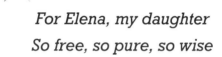

For Elena, my daughter
So free, so pure, so wise

INTRODUCTION

This is a book about courage and surrender. It tells my journey through recent years, where I was taught these lessons in the most perfect ways possible. They did not necessarily come in the most *enjoyable* ways, but were delivered with absolute perfection for my readiness at the time. Life does love us and even though sometimes it can feel like it is all uphill with no sign of hope, we are never fully alone on this journey.

As I learned to trust in the perfection of the lessons, the faster things moved back to ease. To do this, focus had to shift to gratitude (for the perfection of the teachings) and trust (that I would come to see and understand the reason for each lesson in time). The more practiced I became with trusting in the blessings and letting go of the outcome, the more enjoyable and peaceful life became.

So I moved forward one step at a time, in faith, with courage, and always surrendering. In doing so, life has brought me into who I was always here to be. It could not have come about through any other path. I could not be who I am now, a woman in a place of peace, courage, joy, and enthusiasm, without the seemingly impossible hurdles I have overcome.

I share this story with you, dear reader, as a friend. My lessons are universal, even though the specifics are often individual. It is my hope by sharing this story that you, too, will find the strength and courage to surrender to life. There are blessings in whatever challenges unfold on our paths. This story is a tool for opening your eyes to those blessings.

The actual process of writing this book has also been one of courage and surrender. I began writing it when guided, even though I had no knowledge of the ending. In fact, the whole process of this book's evolution was a journey of trust. Occasionally, my life was only a few weeks ahead of the pages I was writing. At other times, I was guided to stop writing for a month or two, here or there. So with courage and conviction, I continued to surrender.

There were themes and longings calling to be shared despite me not having any idea how they would unfold. Yet I continued to write, believing that even if I didn't get the conclusion I hoped for, it would still be the perfect ending for this work of sharing, and more so, for my own path. With such faith, I was only a step ahead of you in knowing how the story was actually going to turn out. (The only change I have made in this whole tale is the name of a dear friend who is mentioned. For his privacy, I changed his name to Jeff.)

I am at peace and in a place of extreme gratitude for where this journey has taken me. Most of all, it has given me the courage to step up and own the role that life has called me to inhabit. It has helped me face my fears, shine my light, and be peaceful with enjoying my life to the fullest, without guilt or self-judgment. It has brought me home into myself.

It is with utmost love and sincerity that I hope it does the same for you.

Life is shaped by the decisions we make.

There are major, well-thought-out ones: Do I move to this town? Do I enter or leave this relationship? Do I speak honestly when I imagine it might create upheaval in my life? Do I choose this method of treatment for an illness?

There are lighthearted decisions: Will I have a cup of chai or fresh juice? Will I wear a purple sweater today or yellow? Will I go for a walk or chill out? Will I call my friend and have a chat now or later?

There are also unconscious ones, both major and lighthearted: I'll take this job because I am too scared to try something new. I'll buy these shoes because my partner won't like them, so I'll feel in control. I'll react this way to that situation because that's how people expect me to. I'll not speak up about my success because I don't want to outshine anyone and attract attention.

Some decisions may start out more as an unconscious desire, rather than a defined decision. Desire is still a choice, though.

So is fear.

So is courage.

2

At some time in my late 20s I made the surprisingly wise decision to always invest my tax refund in myself. I say "surprisingly" because, back then, I was on a path of self-destruction and had such low self-worth that it is quite amazing I could actually honor myself in any way.

One tax refund paid for a camera, as I wanted to sell photos at markets. Another time I walked into a wonderful bookstore and spent a couple of hours filling my basket with wisdom and inspiration. One year I walked over hot coals at a self-empowerment event. Yet another, I took myself off to a meditation retreat, where I loosened all the screws holding the lid of my pain down. So began my conscious path of healing: a journey of courage by listening to my heart, regardless of whatever fears tried to speak more loudly.

The language of the heart is gentle, honest, intelligent, and full of love. Sadly, many people have stopped listening to their yearning. Instead, their shattered hearts have learned to be silent and ever so slowly crumbled. Slight glimmers of hope may have remained for an extended time, ready to bounce back, given the opportunity. Waiting. Waiting. But eventually the voice of the heart is silenced into resignation with a sorrowful sigh, only to be thought of again as the person reflects on their regrets on their deathbed.

Very few can *truly* silence their hearts, though. It sits within, full of wisdom and loving guidance. It calls us forward, somehow drawing us into seeing how beautiful life could really be, if we only have the courage to listen and act. If we do bravely decide to honor that vision, the language of the heart then becomes our most trusted and loyal companion.

3

I t took me a long time to know the language of my heart was talking. A conversation I had with my father helped me recognize that this voice within was *never* going to be silenced. It simply refused, insisting I follow its calling, time and again.

I had been working in a banking job, just another of many that had preceded it. I had worked in locations all around Australia for most of the banks. My roles changed. Methods of transport to and from work changed. Uniforms changed. Not much else really did. The atmosphere in fluorescent-lit offices, the mundane repetition of Monday to Friday, the staff and customer complaints, the pressure for sales targets—it was all the same. My dissatisfaction and eventual heartache at the thought of just going to work did change, though. They increased.

So I quit yet another job. This time I freed myself of the furniture I'd accumulated and traveled back south to visit my parents. "Destination Unknown" from the *Top Gun* soundtrack was my theme song, helping me find romance in the uncertainty of what lay ahead, beyond that visit.

As my father and I drove along a dusty country lane lined with gum trees, the old utility vehicle rattled. Over the bumps and potholes, he asked why I had quit a good job in the bank and what I hoped to achieve by heading off into the unknown.

I didn't know, I told him. I didn't know what to expect. All I did know was that the life of Monday to Friday, nine to five, just didn't fit me. So I was leaving that behind in the hope of finding what did fit.

It was terrifying speaking the words out loud to a man who had ruled my life with criticism and harsh discipline. To have grown into a freethinking adult expressing this new part of myself left butterflies dancing in my stomach. His past manner of controlling me was losing its power. My fear of his usual hostile reaction and rage was subsiding. This conversation was the first indication of that. I felt both nervous and brave, but my heart was speaking more loudly than fear.

I sensed a genuine curiosity in him. This gave me the courage to speak as I did. He then just looked at me with smug amusement and said with a tone of expectant failure, "You'll work it out." Like, you'll come to your senses. You'll come back to a secure job before long.

It was the first time he had ever shown any desire to truly understand me. Even though his response was filled with the lack of hope and expectancy that I'd come to know from him, my yearning began to be defined that very day. I didn't truly know what I wanted. But I sure as anything knew what I didn't.

A month later I was washing dishes on a tropical island on the Great Barrier Reef, as happy as a pig in mud. It became my home for two fabulous years, before a broader world then called me further afield, to experience living in other countries.

My search began in a common place. I knew what was not right, even if I didn't yet know what was. The pain of living wrongly was playing a discordant tune with my heart's rhythm, giving me the courage to start seeking what would feel right.

4

One of the greatest gifts I ever gave to myself was making the decision to start speaking up in my own defense, to stop accepting unkind words from others.

Like many people, I had stayed silent for decades, carrying enormous emotional pain in the process. To do so was both conscious and unconscious.

Consciously, I imagined the turmoil it would create to speak up, to stop old patterns from others in their tracks. Withdrawing inward had always felt like the safest option. That is, until the pain of suppressing things had become too much and I was no longer willing, or more so *able*, to carry it anymore.

My unconscious mind had learned to keep out of the way as a child, to not rock the boat. It had assumed that I deserved to be the venting avenue for anger and cruelty from some members of my family, that it was okay to take the load on. It had decided that a mediocre, quiet life was better than dealing with pain and breaking free.

Turmoil certainly appeared during these chapters of change. Great fear and uncertainty were triggered. Others also had to learn new ways to associate with me. I was not the same person as before. So the old games carried less and less significance, until they merely became an opportunity for me to grow in compassion for others when I saw the old ways reappear.

My own fear and resistance in learning to give myself such kindness, however, was so fixed that it took sliding into a painfully dark period of depression to shatter it. Decades of pain, abuse, self-judgment, and absolute heartache rose to the surface. It had to come out if I was to be truly healed. Out it came—in bucket loads of tears for months on end.

Life had blessed me with an ideal scenario for such release. I was surrounded by nature, living in a little cottage by a running creek. The natural rhythms and wildlife nurtured my soul as my thoughts of myself and others gradually shifted toward more loving directions.

Given that time and isolation, the potential I had dared to glimpse inside for many years was now shaping the new me. I was breaking through the shell of conformity and conditioning from my past. A new person was emerging, full of hope and, eventually, great optimism.

I was also learning how to love me, how to treat myself with immense kindness in both action *and* thought. The lessons became enjoyable. They were gentle. I gradually stopped seeing them as something to be frightened of. Every conscious choice toward self-kindness helped new habits form, whether soaking in the bath on a Tuesday afternoon or not joining a conversation that might disempower me. There was now an obvious purpose in the learning: to walk more freely from emotional pain. As courage increased to honor my own needs and desires, guilt and shame grew weaker. It was actually okay to steer my life toward happiness.

Going through depression allowed tears that needed to be released throughout my life, and hadn't been, to finally do so. Drop by drop, walls around the heart washed away, allowing it to grow stronger. The changes were gradual, carried forward on a moment-to-moment basis through letting go, making kinder choices toward myself, and having my own permission to just be in the moment, whatever it may be.

If my feelings came up against resistance, when old ways feared letting kindness through, the heart waited, as love does, with patience and gentleness. When it was ready to open up just a little bit more again, love would seep in and heal yet another tender part of myself.

In deciding to speak up, there were many habits and triggers to undo. With increasing practice of self-kindness, I continued to improve, until the patterns were shattered completely. I no longer attracted the situations that had always brought me so much pain. Relationships either improved and became more respectful, or they fell away completely.

My load grew lighter. Re-entering the world again was not scary anymore. It was exciting, with new hopes rising up and out. One step at a time a fresh chapter began. A new person emerged. Courage held my hand as I ventured forth into a different world. It was a place that I didn't yet know consciously but one that the deepest parts, the secret parts of my heart, had always known and longed for.

Having braved the storm and its fallout, having come through to the soothing love of the sun on the other side, I felt quietly empowered. As the lessons in self-love continued, I walked on gently, sometimes slightly tentatively, but with faith that it was all going to be okay after all.

It was time to learn how to step up and own my role in this life. With a lighter load I answered the call to keep moving forward. Life was enticing me to know who this remarkable person within truly was. (We are *all* remarkable.)

My potential was truly limited only by thoughts of myself. These were shaped by many factors. But every small decision and action I could make in kindness toward myself was a loving step toward that potential. This possibility was not about achievements in society, though those may have come. It was about living in true peace within—and with that, all of life could change so beautifully.

5

As the haze of depression lifted, life continued to improve daily. New opportunities for writing arrived, with my work growing rapidly on a global scale. I became emotionally strong enough to create a songwriting program for some disadvantaged women in my local area. To experience a sense of capability again was gratifying.

An even larger call was also coming through. It was the desire to be a parent. By now I was into my 40s and previously had let go of the idea of becoming a mum. Any former relationships I had been in were consistent in that the partners had addictions. Further into the past, I'd also had my own habit of regular pot smoking, though that was now well gone.

With the addictions in partners, I had justified the acceptance of each situation to myself. This one was an alcoholic, but at least he wasn't violent or aggressive. This one was a daily pot smoker, but at least he didn't drink, and so on. Several years were spent seeing the potential in partners before realizing they were not seeing it in themselves. Several years were also spent not recognizing my own low self-worth that justified these types of relationships. Still, I was growing and patterns were changing.

I was single at the time. I had needed to be anyway. Being gifted with that time in solitude to break free within myself was the greatest of all. I enjoyed single life. Independence worked for me. Yet the longing to become a parent continued to grow stronger, seemingly out of nowhere.

Foster parenting was an option I had considered, but not as yet in such presence to put in an application. It floated by. Life was telling me otherwise. My body screamed to hurry up. The feeling of a little girl waiting in the background became more prominent. So did the hope of joining with a partner in a relationship.

As the doors of change and opportunity continued opening, welcoming me into my new life after depression, I met a man with whom I became friends. In time, we became lovers. Two months after that, we intentionally conceived a baby. I was 44 years old. The call to become pregnant had been so strong that it hadn't crossed my mind I could be unsuccessful. Luckily I lived in a world where inner guidance spoke louder than media statistics about possibilities.

One evening I was sitting around a campfire, chatting with a friend. My partner and I had made love that afternoon. As I relaxed in the camping chair, enjoying the warmth of the roaring fire and the incredible blanket of stars above, I felt a moment of faintness. Then came a rush of love through every cell in my body. It was impossible to ignore. A pinpoint of a star flashed brightly in my mind as euphoria flooded through me. It was *incredible*, as my body voluntarily loosened and relaxed, surrendering to the rush. And then it was gone, just like that.

The fire continued to burn as it was. The stars continued to shimmer. But I smiled inwardly. Conception had just occurred. I knew it. I just knew it. The conversation continued, but my heart was leaping in joy too much for me to remain present. *I am going to be a mother!* To top that off, I had already shared such a connection with my child that she had let me know she had arrived. *Welcome, little one. Stay safe in there. I love you already.*

Life took on new meaning. I had lived more than a quarter of a century of adulthood and experienced much in that time. Freedom certainly had not been wasted on me, thank goodness. But now it was not going to be about me. There was a precious, divine little being to consider.

The pregnancy was confirmed six weeks later. By then, I was already naturally experiencing life as a mother and seeing things *much* more clearly. It was like a haze had lifted—one I hadn't even realized existed. Out of compassion, I had made a lot of excuses for certain dynamics within the friendship and relationship with my partner. Now that I was a mother and further time was unfolding, I viewed life through the clearest eyes I had ever known. What I saw were enormous warnings and signposts offering vastly different choices.

It became clear to me that for the safety and wellbeing of both the baby and myself, I actually had to leave the relationship with my partner. The child and I were going to spend our lives in a volatile existence otherwise. It could not be risked.

Although the decision took courage and brought significant sadness, my job was to provide a healthy and safe environment for the child. Further events unfolded, insisting I had made the right choice. Another decision then followed. It was time to return to my home region.

It had been 27 years since I had lived there long-term. There had been periods in between my roaming when I had ended up back under my parents' roof. But I'd never gone back with any sense or intention of staying. The call to return was now so strong that I could not have denied it if I tried.

Obviously, the thought of physical and emotional support for my baby from my own mother was enticing. I also wanted my child to know her grandparents, so this was the best way to enable that.

My relationship with my own grandmother had shaped me in a significant and positive way. It was important for me that my own babe would be given the opportunity to form a similar bond with her grandmother. So I found gratitude in the gift of time and opportunity that I was creating in regard to that.

There was also my financial situation to consider. To me, money had always been a tool for doing, not for having. Whenever I'd had any savings accumulated in the past, my thoughts were always, *Where can I go now?* Experiences were always far more important than belongings. Several years of irregular work as a caregiver and a nomadic lifestyle certainly didn't provide me with financial security either. So through that period of depression a year or so earlier, when I was not actually capable of working, things became somewhat challenging to say the least.

I had been in such a terribly low place that I'd had to accept food vouchers from charity networks to survive. It had been an enormous lesson in learning to receive. It was challenging to master, but how could I allow in any true goodness if I didn't? I was also learning how to be kinder to me. So I did my best not to judge myself too harshly for the situation I had (unintentionally) created.

Things had improved immensely since then, thankfully. In addition to teaching songwriting, I had finished writing my first full-length book. I'd also been performing music shows for young children. Work had taken off. I was in a much healthier place and still on the up-and-up. But until I could afford my own place, living with my parents as an extended family was the best option.

My parents and I adapted as best we could and fell into our own groove together. There were some very special times between us while the baby continued to grow within. Mum and I grew more into our relationship as women every day, no longer just as mother and daughter. Walking around the streets of the small country village, with magnificent mountains only a few miles away, hours of memorable conversations unfolded. When walking became waddling, the conversations became shorter, as did the distances walked. The subjects discussed remained just as rich.

While I was certainly grateful for the room and comfortable home to live in, there were challenges adjusting, especially after having experienced independent living for a couple of decades. The relationship my father and I had shared until recent years had been tumultuous. His uncontrollable anger was terrifying to me as a child and antagonistic to me as a teenager. Decades of criticism from him had done immense damage. Even with his intimidatingly brusque manner, he could not demand my respect—that was something he had to earn.

In coming to terms with my own healing, however, our relationship had improved in recent years. I had learned to speak up, resulting in him learning to treat me differently, more respectfully. Time, illness, and experience had also mellowed him considerably. I grew in compassion and recognized his efforts, hence doing my best to create kindness in our interactions rather than avoidance. We were both trying and did pretty well considering the immense pain that I had lived with, based on my interpretations of our relationship. When it came to my pregnancy, he could not have been a kinder dad.

Mum and I had always been close, though there were struggles happening within me regarding losing my independence. I was living in another woman's home and had to respect her ways and her insistence in doing so much for me at a time when I wanted to do much more for myself. It wasn't going to be forever, though. I knew that. So I focused on the gift of time, feeling sure that in future years I would look back on that chapter as the special blessing it was for us all.

In the meantime my body shape altered daily. The babe moved around. My size increased. The time of further change grew inevitably closer. I was almost 45 years old and about to become a first-time mum. The final months were spent staying cool in a comfortable home as the summer sun scorched down outside.

I was at peace with the decisions I had made, with no regrets in having left the relationship. Life's signposts had been too clear for me to overlook. Each time they guided me, beyond room for any doubt, I could not reason with argument. There were simply occasions in life when the signposts were too glaringly obvious to dare ignore. Leaving the relationship had bittersweetly been one of those times.

On a soul level, I was still grateful to the child's father for the experiences his role had brought to my life. He was always going to be her biological father, too. I would not stand in the way of that, assuring the wellbeing of the child in the process.

For now, though, life as a solo mum was about to begin. The due date approached, then passed. More than another week dragged on. Then her time arrived. My baby was coming. As life would have it, the arrival of my largest work success thus far had decided to come at the very same time.

6

efore you are a parent, it is easy to imagine the scenario of becoming one. The reality is quite a contrast. Certainly I had never imagined experiencing the pain of contractions late at night in my hospital bed, while fielding interviews from international journalists. But that was my reality. Instead of the success of my work or, more important, the arrival of my baby being an exciting thought, I was overwhelmed with pressure.

All my years of hard work were finally paying off. It had taken 14 years to become an overnight success. My book was gaining wonderful momentum. This brought media opportunities to me—from left, right, and center. Questions regarding translation rights also poured in. I had worked hard for this, drawing on an immense amount of courage to stay focused on getting my message to its audience. The success I deserved was indeed manifesting. But rather than riding the wave of excitement I'd imagined would come with it, I experienced heartache.

My baby was coming into the world, her willingness to join me on the outside making itself more apparent by the hour. I wanted to feel present for this experience more than anything. This time would never come again. There would never be another birth, another child. My body had blessed me with this one, very healthy, pregnancy. I didn't need to tempt fate and try for more children, particularly as I was entering parenthood as a solo late-in-life mum.

As I turned off my phone and computer near midnight, the prayer I sent out was clear: *I need help with my book, and I need it now. Please!*

The following morning I was advised my baby's head was in the wrong position and an emergency cesarean was needed. Although a part of me was definitely saddened that it was not to be a natural birth, I was not willing to risk my little one's life. A few hours later I was in surgery.

There were students and interns watching. I hadn't minded, I said. My mum was there, too. As they prepared me for the procedure, the conversation I heard was about how bad the car-parking situation was at the hospital. It was a lively, animated conversation with hardly anyone actually acknowledging the reverence of the moment, of a babe about to enter the world.

You've got to be joking, I thought. All I wanted was silence and beauty. That was difficult enough in a room with nearly a dozen people and bright surgery lights. But conversations about car parking? Seriously? Again, it was time for me to send a very clear and immediate prayer: *Shut them up.* Now. *Please!*

Instantly, the conversation died off and focus shifted to the procedure and the somewhat enormous baby being found within my womb. "Thank you," I breathed to God and my spiritual helpers, fortunately tuned into the reverence of the occasion. "Thank you."

I hated the whole procedure as far as having my baby pulled out, her cord being snipped immediately rather than delayed, and her being weighed and wrapped, all before we were able to experience skin-to-skin contact. But I had still brought a healthy, gorgeous little girl into the world.

When they laid Elena on my chest, we just looked at each other at first. The wisdom in her eyes blew me away instantly. While losing myself in them, all I could do was whisper, "Hi," ever so softly. Then gently I smiled and kissed her head. "Hi," I repeated in a whisper. Forever I was bound to this little being, one who had waited so patiently all those years to enter my life.

The following morning in a busy hospital room, my prayer for help was answered. The managing director of my favorite book publisher phoned and offered me an international publishing deal. It was as if I were skating in a dream and they simply decided to skate along beside me. There was no jolt, other than some tears of relief and gratitude, just a smooth transition supporting the next chapter of my life. When I left the hospital five days later, it was with a precious baby and a publishing contract. Talk about timing.

Life can change so quickly. It was indeed blessing my efforts. And in the meantime, I was continuing to learn how to open up and allow myself to receive the increasing bounties flowing my way.

7

With the publishing deal came sufficient funds for me to support my daughter and myself, provided I kept our living simple. That was the lifestyle that fitted me best anyway, so it was not a sacrifice to make. My needs were quite few. In time, the success of the book also brought me a down payment for our own house.

Until then, we were still under my parents' roof. They were already grandparents and adored their roles. Now both were incredibly clucky and loving with their latest grandchild, my little Elena. Mum went into overdrive and kissed her about two hundred times a day, no exaggeration. Dad would call me in to look at her when she was sleeping during the day, to reassure him that she was breathing. Sometimes I would walk past our bedroom door to find him just standing there, looking at her. It was an incredibly bonding time for us all.

There were also times, increasingly, when I longed to be more independent and have a little more control over the parenting of my child. But again, I tried to let go and find the blessings in the situation. The search for a home to purchase had begun. My mortgage application was approved—something that was quite amazing considering my previous few years financially. Life continued to support me in this way.

What was becoming impossible to ignore following Elena's arrival into the world, however, were the lingering aches in my hands and feet, particularly in the mornings. Initially it felt like a bit of an inconvenience, like a flu that sets you off balance a bit but you know will pass. I kept waiting for the aches to go. Eventually I had to admit to myself that they were actually getting worse.

My local doctor, who had known the family for years, was a darling person—full of cheek but incredibly wise in his profession.

When I explained how I was feeling, he asked several questions with a knowing tone and then sent me for blood tests.

Sitting on the lounge at home a couple of days later, with my babe at the breast, I answered the phone to hear him say that the tests had confirmed his suspicions. In a solemn tone he advised me I had rheumatoid arthritis. He insisted I come in to see him the following day as a matter of urgency.

Although I had a friend in England who was living with rheumatoid arthritis (RA) and knew she had to have several joints replaced over the years, the enormity of my own situation didn't really sink in. I figured I could knock it on the head in no time with a healthy diet and positive attitude. Oh, how simple that would have been! When I had experienced depression and almost taken my life, I'd figured things could never become as challenging again. I had survived the biggest test possible. Little did I know the strength I'd developed in surviving that chapter was merely a trial run for all that lay ahead.

8

The first step was to visit my doctor again. He advised me of my options regarding medication, all of which he emphatically supported. His urgency and passion about this were impossible to ignore. Painting pictures of my life without the medications was something he did remarkably well.

Yet I didn't feel at all guided to go down that path. The medications had a list of potential side effects 10 miles long, and I would have to cease breast-feeding. Elena was only a couple of months old, and there was no way I was doing that. I was also living an incredibly clean lifestyle—a healthy diet and zero alcohol or drugs. The thought of putting chemotherapy medication into my system, which is what it was in a milder dose, was horrifying and too toxic to consider. I couldn't wrap my head around it.

I researched as much as I could about the disease, becoming increasingly overwhelmed when reading forums of other RA sufferers. I made the decision to stop visiting those forums as everyone there appeared bonded by the disease, a situation I had no desire to be in.

Instead I turned to researching success stories. They were few and far between, but they kept me going—those and my own determination to see the lessons as a gift. There was no doubt in my mind that despite the increasing pain, there was healing on offer, too. I would embrace that experience as best I could.

Through the Vipassana meditation path that I had followed for several years, I had learned to tolerate pain at incredible levels. When you sit in silence from 4:30 A.M. to 9:00 P.M. for 10 consecutive days with just a few hours' break each day, you tend to experience and release a lot of physical and emotional pain alongside the blissful experiences.

With repeated courses, I learned to observe the pain rather than react to it. Likewise for the euphoria I experienced. The theory was based on the Buddha's teachings: All suffering is caused by craving and aversion. The technique allowed me to experience that firsthand. If I started craving the good feelings, they went away. If I feared the pain, it increased. So I learned to observe them for what they were, transient experiences (as is all of life). Then neither had power over me and I became a more equanimous observer—neither longing for good nor averting learning (often perceived as negative). I learned to simply observe what is, opening myself up to a much smoother life. The less resistance or attachment I had, the more naturally and gently life flowed my way. Above all, the more present I became.

It was through the firsthand experience of the pain while meditating that, in time, I developed those tools in regular life too. They became a natural part of my thinking process. The learning never stopped, of course. So there were still plenty of lapses into humanness and vulnerability that included fear and longing. Generally, though, this way of viewing life assisted in so many aspects of day-to-day living. I learned to become more detached from outcomes, but more peaceful and loving in the process.

It was through this approach that I first managed the pain becoming increasingly present—trying to stay detached and observing it without too much aversion. Occasionally I would take a very mild painkiller, even though that idea made me cringe at the time since I was so anti-medication. Instead I usually tried to observe the pain and trust that it would pass. Sure enough, it would come and go in waves. When it was gone, I focused on remembering the feeling of wellness as best I could.

As well as writing, another creative outlet I loved was songwriting. With the publishing advance I was able to record my second album. It had been five years since I had recorded and released my first, back when the path of being a singer/songwriter was much more prominent in my life. Not having had the funds to record the second album in the time since, I had a backlog of songs I'd written that were longing to be shared.

I loved the fact that life was now calling me onto the author's path rather than continuing as a singer/songwriter. The author's lifestyle suited my quiet nature much better—but there were still messages in the existing songs that deserved release.

So in between breast-feeding, changing nappies, and exhaustion, I managed to record my album, *Songs for the Soul*. I was thrilled to experience the sense of completion that followed. As motherhood was now my current priority, I felt fine to be releasing some of my music time, knowing that the album was done. For years, including up until two days before Elena was born, I had played my guitar almost every day.

Three days after the recording process was complete, an absolute *inferno* of pain set into my hands, crippling their movement enormously. I was unable to tell if the fingers could actually move or not, as the raging heat was too distracting to feel a thing beyond it. If someone told me they had lifted my skin off while I slept, filled my hands and fingers with glowing coals from a fire, then sealed the skin back up, I would have believed them. Comprehending just how intensely my hands burned, without an obvious fire, was beyond me.

Despite that same pain continuing in waves, it took another couple of weeks to accept the fact that I couldn't actually play my beloved guitar anymore. The intensity of burning meant that any unnecessary movement was impossible. So the instrument sat in its stand, waiting for my caress and for our bond. Each night as the moonlight filtered into my room, I would see its silhouette, sitting, waiting. Finally, as my little girl slept soundly, I began to face the truth of my current situation. After staring at the ceiling for ages, pondering the actual enormity, I rolled over and sobbed myself to sleep.

The following morning, with teary eyes and a broken heart, I put my guitar into its case and removed it from sight. Looking out the window at a sparrow singing, I prayed, "Please let this be worth it."

At that particular moment, my sadness didn't actually manage the strength for hope. I allowed it to be what it was—a moment of fragility and utter heartbroken sadness.

9

The home situation began shifting after some months, when I found a house to purchase. Despite living independently and afar for those couple of decades, a nostalgic part of me had always longed for some sort of warm, united, and loving family unit. As the intention in moving back to my home region had been to be nearer to my mum, whom I had always missed when living elsewhere, I chose a nearby location only five minutes down the road from my parents' home.

While the period of legalities and settlement was happening for the house, I was blessed with a trip to England to promote my book and begin my speaking career. With little Elena worn in a carrier, snuggly wrapped into the front of my body, off we went with a smile and a wave. It felt wonderful to be out of the village and back into the broader world. Mine had shrunk so much over the previous year or so.

The dose of travel and the melting pot of humanity found at airports and in London were a balm to my soul. I felt alive again and connected to an old part of myself that had been lost. Through the years of caring for dying people, then my chosen withdrawal from society while depressed, followed by living with my parents in a tiny rural village, I had somehow lost one of the parts of myself I most loved.

The traveler, the adventurer, the free-spirited woman who had been such a part of me for so long, now insisted on surfacing. Although I had little Elena with me the whole time, I experienced a long-forgotten feeling: the freedom of independence.

Walking, particularly long distances, had always been a particular love of mine, along with swimming. During the first week in London, I walked as many streets as I could. Sometimes Elena was in the stroller, but usually she was strapped to me. We fell into our own groove together, and the bond of mother and daughter strengthened in a way I had been longing for. She was an amazing little traveler, smiling at strangers and melting hearts wherever we went.

One night while Elena was asleep, my hands began searing in pain like I had not yet known. It was as if someone had thrown a tin of petrol onto the existing daily inferno. A hurricane also blew, adding power to the intensity. As it increased, I closed the bathroom door behind me and proceeded to weep uncontrollably. Holding up my hands and looking at them, I sobbed at the heart-wrenching loss of health and ability. Sliding to the floor, I leaned against the bathtub. My hands, my precious, talented, essential hands, what was happening? Heat raged until I could no longer even lift them from the unbearable weight of pain. "Dear God," I prayed. "Please send me some help. I am not strong enough to handle this level of pain. Dear God. *Please help me.*"

Eventually, the intensity did lessen a little, releasing me into a troubled sleep full of emotional and physical exhaustion. The following morning my first stop was at a pharmacy, where I requested the strongest painkillers for RA possible while still breast-feeding. The rest of the trip was spent watching the clock, longing for the next four hours to roll around so I could take another dose. Tiredness from constant painkillers began limiting me. Even our walks suffered as they could no longer be for hours on end.

Luckily we were accommodated a short walk from Kensington Gardens, so at least we could enjoy some time there. I sat against a huge tree, watching so many seemingly healthy people pass by. Elena happily ate her mushy food then fell asleep at my breast, the dear little babe. I felt a sense of peace in the gardens. Mother Earth had always been successful in nurturing my heart when aching. She did the same then.

I knew enough to understand the vicious cycle of painkillers— that in time, the more you take, the more you need, and, ultimately, you create more pain through a process where you can't win. But I had to deal with the current situation. The disease was giving me a lesson in presence like none before. *One day at a time*, I told myself.

I attended to the work commitments, including a quick trip to the Netherlands. It should have been wonderful. Like my English publishers, the Dutch ones were lovely people and truly made me feel welcome. Now, though, the pain had decided to visit my feet. The cobbled streets of Amsterdam and the narrow stairs in the beautiful historic hotel felt like thorns. I longed to be back in my London hotel room, resting, *forever*. Movement and exertion began to feel too hard. Thank goodness I had already walked so much in London, though that felt like little consolation.

With crippling hands and agonizing feet, we somehow made it back to Australia. At the airports and on the flights, I had to ask other people to unbuckle the carrier I held Elena in whenever she wanted out. The strength in my hands and fingers had reduced so much that I was becoming dependent on others in small ways. Lifting Elena also had to be done with my lower arms instead of my hands. But she adapted, as children do.

We had to exit our plane in Singapore while they cleaned it. Friendly airport officials found me a stroller and up sat little Elena, full of wonder and joy. She smiled at people to such a degree that a crowd formed around us. I couldn't walk on. With a mass of curls and big beautiful eyes, Elena was as pretty as a baby can be. At one stage, we had about 30 people crowded around us, all patiently waiting their turn to touch her and get a smile. Elena obliged perfectly with absolutely no limitations.

While all of this was happening, the tenderness in my feet started to become crippling. I desperately wanted to collapse on the floor. It took great persistence to disperse the crowd in the most pleasant way possible. We returned to the waiting lounge so I could sit, but the pain raged on. By the time we boarded the plane I was hobbling like a sickly 90-year-old. That was the day I lost my smooth, bouncy gait. An ongoing limp had arrived.

Mum and Dad's house was a welcome help on my return. Elena and I fell into bed and a deep jet-lagged sleep. On waking, I easily accepted Mum's dedication and longing for time with my little girl. My bond with Elena was now sealed in a way that brought me peace. We had enjoyed such quality time together while away. And in a short time, we would be moving into our own home. Settlement date on the property purchase was drawing closer. I could get on with properly being the mother I wanted to be.

That was my hope anyway.

10

Sentimentality was obviously a part of me. Despite not enjoying many aspects of my childhood and not staying in the relationship with Elena's biological father, I was still searching for peace with my concept of family. I loved the coastal regions. I loved the rain. Most of the things I loved were not available in the region to which I had returned. Yet it was without a doubt that I had to come back.

In hindsight, I'd probably had RA for some years. It seemed to be triggered only when I was back visiting family. My shoulder would freeze up. Or once, my hand was so hot I couldn't use it to change gears in my van. I'd had to reach my other hand across to do it. Sometimes my feet swelled too. A friend who lived in a nearby town was a talented body worker and healer. So I would visit her and be gifted with a treatment through whatever modality she was guided to do on the day. It always helped, and we would laugh about me having "hometown-itis" again. When I would return to whatever region I was living in, away from there, the symptoms never accompanied me, so I would forget about them.

I accepted there was more healing to do associated with family and my home region, but I hadn't dwelled on it. As I moved into my new home, there was now no denying or escaping it. On top of that, the disease had risen so much to the surface that moving away was not going to subdue it. It was time to face the situation.

There had never been a challenge in my life that I didn't find a blessing in. It was the only way I could approach upheaval— to trust that in the big picture, it was all perfect. During strong moments, I drew inspiration from various teachers and from within. *Only good will come from this situation*, I told myself. There would be gifts of learning through this journey and, damn it, I was going to find them! But well before that I had to reach a place of facing the reality that this was not an overnight thing.

The shock was difficult. One moment I was strong and healthy, and now I had seemingly no control over the demise of my health. The loss of physical freedom and independence was almost as unbearable as the constant pain. Although I immediately went into healing mode as best I could through diet and attitude, the symptoms increased.

RA, particularly early on, rages best in evenings and mornings, though it doesn't actually let up during the night either. An inability to gain any restful sleep, in between the babe waking all through the night for feeding and my pain, left me in a state of haze that became my reality for far longer than anticipated.

The disease is a bit like the old arcade game *Pac-Man*. There are two hungry little gremlins. They each choose a side of the body, then say to each other, "Where shall we go now?" The other thinks about it for a second and replies, "Well, we haven't eaten the knees for a while—let's go there." Then off they go, eating away at any health in that region. Both sides of the body were affected, but from hour to hour, it was impossible to know where the pain was going to arise next.

The difference of one centimeter in angling a particular part of the body was the determining factor for sleep. Just as I would find the comfortable position despite the raging pain and try to sleep, the gremlins would head off somewhere else. Now instead of the hands, it would be the ankles, or elbows, shoulders, jaw, fingers, wrists. The cotton sheet became too large a weight to bear on my toes. I found I had joints I didn't even realize had existed, particularly when the disease moved into my rib cage.

Sleep, what I needed most, was unattainable. Each morning I woke and slowly made my way to the bathroom. Confidence was sliding away as I hobbled along, unsteady and increasingly terrified. My greatest fear was I would fall and not be able to get up. This fear escalated into family or officials taking Elena away, stating I couldn't look after her.

I held on to furniture as I moved about the house, once standing motionless for quite a few minutes, wondering if I *could* actually walk the three steps needed to get to the next piece. It was terrifying, wobbling on unsteady feet, not daring to lift either in case the remaining one couldn't support me.

Life was teaching me honesty in its most raw form. I could no longer pretend, especially to myself, that I was okay.

11

onths rolled by, of much the same. People kept telling me how quickly time goes when you have a young child. Not for me. It felt as though time stood still. Every day felt like a year. Every morning felt like waking from a bad dream only to realize it wasn't a dream.

Weight had begun falling off. I'd put on quite a bit when pregnant, so I didn't mind this initially. But as it continued to disappear, so did my strength. Most of my energy was going into overcoming the raging pain.

A haircut followed a few months later. My shoulders were in too much pain to lift my elbows more than four or five inches out from my chest. Even on good days when they would lift, my hands couldn't properly hold a hairbrush and my wrists didn't have the strength to pull a comb or brush through long hair. So for the first time in years, I had short hair.

My wrists felt their demise from the disease well before everywhere else. Often the weight of my own hands was too heavy for them to bear. I would have to just sit. That's it. Sit. Do nothing other than watch my little girl discovering her world. I'd sing or talk but not be able to use my hands at all. Then the gremlins would move on to somewhere else and up I'd get. Or at least I would try.

Getting up and down had become a nightmare. Media regarding body image had influenced me when I was a young woman, like it unfortunately does to most young women. I had hated my strong thighs. Thankfully over the years I had learned to let go of that and treat my body with more loving thoughts. Now I was extremely grateful for the strong thighs that enabled me to get up and down. Without them, life would have been even more restrictive.

There was a rocking chair that I breast-fed Elena in. Sometimes we'd just sit there talking. She was growing fast and had much to say, even if I couldn't understand most of it. The momentum from the rocking often helped me stand. On one particular day, even that didn't help. After a few efforts rocking back and forth to rise, I sighed, resigned. Sitting for another couple of moments, I asked aloud to no one, "How am I going to get up from this chair?" My dear little girl then came over and tried to pull me up. It broke my heart and gave me the determination to rise on my own, despite the pain.

There came a time when I had to admit that I no longer had the strength to breast-feed Elena. She was now 17 months old and incredibly robust for her age. It had always been my hope to wean naturally, to allow the child to determine her own time. Had she wanted to continue until she was five, I wouldn't have cared. Society's opinion was not a part of my concern regarding my parenting choices. My health, however, was.

Elena was incredibly intuitive and understanding over coming days. "Please, Mummy," she would ask while gently trying to lift my shirt. With tears in my eyes, I would shake my head, gently saying sorry. My grief was overwhelming. That bond would never return, and I hated the disease for forcing this process before our time. Elena began resting her head on my tummy while drinking from a bottle, always holding my breast at the same time. We both had our own versions of letting go.

The tenderness in my feet was awful. It was also becoming somewhat more consistent. It felt as if a horse wearing its metal shoes had stomped on the top of both feet repeatedly with full force. The balls and heels of my feet felt as though someone had taken to them with a hammer, over and over. Yet I tried to walk. In time, any uneven surface was impossible. I lived in sandals and was increasingly limited to flat surfaces. Even grass was too painful to walk on. The slightest bump or tiny slope was just too hard.

Dependence on Mum increased, as I didn't have the energy to go to town more than necessary. It was also a town where I was known. Not because I was Bronnie Ware, the author. My family had lived there a long time, so local people always saw me as the daughter or sister of someone they knew. I couldn't go to town without running into someone I recognized through association. It didn't take long to grow weary of the questions regarding my walking. I didn't need the attention. I was exhausted enough. Mum would regularly drop by and shop for me instead.

As my work was doing well, I was blessed to be able to continue working from home. The seeds I had sown over the previous decade and more were now sprouting enough for me to pay my bills and keep the roof over our heads. I felt very blessed. I wasn't so cashed up yet that I could go, "Whoopee," and travel the world first class, but I had enough income flowing in to provide for our life.

Even so, there were rare occasions when I had to venture out for work. Once, I headed down to Melbourne to speak at a writers' workshop. I was excited by the opportunity—partly to reconnect with lots of positive people through my work and partly to have a weekend away. My parents were delighted to have Elena all to themselves. I knew I would long for her, but I was too exhausted to keep going.

The first night in the hotel, the temptation of a long soak in the bath was too much for me. As the warm water rushed in, my throbbing feet anticipated relief with urgency. Once the water was right, I climbed in. Unfortunately, as my knees were no longer working right, I ended up sliding down into the bath rather than gently sitting down. I had a feeling I might be in strife getting out, but the water was so wonderful that I just let go and enjoyed it. It had been so long since I had relaxed at such a level. No one needed me. The bathroom was all mine. I lay back and closed my eyes as the water soothed my frail, aching body and weary heart.

Then came the time to get out—and I couldn't. I attempted to a few times with the water still in, but gave up and released the plug. Still, my hands, wrists, and elbows did not have enough strength to propel me up. My knees wouldn't bend enough to get my feet under me to stand, not that I could without support from my hands anyway. The bath mat lay nearby, so I put it inside the bath to offer some grip and stop me sliding as I tried again. That didn't work either.

After *several* repeated efforts, tears of frustration started to surface. Before long they increased, until I was sitting in the empty bath crying at full volume. It was the first time I'd been able to truly let go on that primal level. I cried for everything and anything in frustration and utter heartache. I cried, sobbed, and prayed. It was a well-overdue process of emptying out through tears.

After what seemed like forever, I was indeed as empty as the bath I sat in—and still the predicament remained. I had no idea how I was going to get out. Strangely, there was an emergency button by the toilet. I could see it, but it was well out of reach, as was my phone. Reassessing the situation, I knew there was no choice. I *had* to find my own way out of the bath.

It took everything I had, but somehow I did it. I slid about a few times first, ending up lying on my side in the bath with hands that could not get me upright immediately. But with fierce determination, I eventually lifted my elbows up the side enough to hinge a foot over. Once that leg blindly found solid ground, my upper body somehow followed. It wasn't graceful, but it was successful.

Lying on the big, comfortable bed after that, I easily made the decision that was to be my last bath for the time being. Another freedom slipped further away.

As heavy eyelids seduced me into sleep, a prayer escaped my thoughts. *Please tell me what else I can do. What am I missing?*

My dream that night remained elusive.

12

Determined to find the blessings through the disease, I had to try to understand it. If I had attracted it subconsciously, then on a soul level, there must be healing on offer for me, too. I couldn't reason with any other thinking.

RA is one of many autoimmune diseases where the theory is the immune system is attacking healthy cells. In the case of RA, the attack is on the lining of the joints. If considering the current medical facts, the bottom line was that I was attacking myself. However, increasing evidence was coming through that all autoimmune diseases were actually linked to the gut and digestion.

There was a lot of learning to do, which I embraced as best as possible. Once it became evident there was no easy way over this, I began the journey through it instead. Never once did I choose to call it *my* disease, though. It was *a* disease, one that was here to teach me, but one I would never claim attachment to. While it was certainly shaping my journey, I didn't want it to determine my identity. For that reason, it was quite some time before I made it known to most people I actually had the disease at all.

A thing about pain—a good thing—is that it allowed me to cry. It was forcing me to. In the process, it gave permission for emotional pain to surface, too. There was no true separation of the two anyway. Without emotional pain, there would be no physical pain, no disease to heal in the first place. Everyone has emotional pain to heal regardless of whether it surfaces as disease or not. Sometimes it will surface through other trauma.

With life throwing such an enormous curveball my way, it was actually throwing me a loving call home—a call that offered me the opportunity to grow more into who I was truly meant to be.

Going within the body, I couldn't get much deeper than the bones. So with the pain surfacing from there, I figured life was calling me to heal the very deepest reaches of emotional pain.

I'd thought I had healed so much in the past through the conscious journey of personal growth I had already embarked upon. Topping that off with the transformative time through depression, I was certainly not the person I used to be. I had found a new level of kindness toward myself—and a much more peaceful existence.

It felt as if life was not only making sure I understood and practiced self-care, but that I lived and breathed it with every single part of my being. If I had attracted a disease where I was attacking myself, then on some level I had to find that habit within and heal it.

There were various great books that offered suggestions for the metaphysical causes of the disease. While I took them into consideration, my own guidance was clear enough to find my own answers. The heart was talking loudly. With each episode of intensity, it was not only the physical pain or frustration of decreasing abilities that brought tears. It was the permission for release. As I let the torrent pour, emotions surfaced from the deepest parts of my being. While I was crying in physical pain, it also shifted invisibly to include whatever matters of the heart were still yearning for love.

Three conclusions became obvious, though they all encompassed the one healing direction.

I had to learn forgiveness toward myself.

I felt guilty for being too happy.

And I had upper-limit problems.

Life was trying to bless me with an amazing life, but I had not yet reached a place where I could truly allow it to flow. I was trying. I was certainly letting more flow to me than I used to. But major healing rarely happens overnight. There are so many layers, *so* many! I had healed plenty, but now I was into the bones of my healing, in the truest sense.

Realizing I had to forgive myself was actually a heck of an eye-opener. I had felt I was already treating myself with kind thoughts and gentleness. When the guidance surfaced within that I needed to forgive myself, it took me aback. "What for?" I questioned.

Whoa! What a question that turned out to be. The answers started pouring out, and the path to my true healing finally began. I looked at my crying face in the mirror and lovingly apologized.

Without any conscious intention, my first apology was to the little girl within me, who had so badly wanted to believe in the goodness of life. Instead, through avoidance of further ridicule, abuse, and cruelty from others, she had learned to withdraw—anything to avoid being noticed and attracting condemnation. I was sorry for leaving it so long to courageously speak up in self-protection. I was sorry I had allowed my life to be so shaped by the ignorant opinions of others.

Apologies poured out to my body, too. I was sorry for the way I had treated it in earlier times. There had been years of awfully critical thoughts directed at it just because it wasn't the shape I wanted it to be. I had indulged in numerous drugs along the way, particularly in my 20s, and had expected my body to carry on. I'd hated myself so much that I had also been a heavy cigarette smoker in earlier years—a thought that grew to repulse me. My poor but loyal body had endured extensive cruelty from me. Tears of apology continued.

There had also been an addiction to pornography at one stage, when I was in such a shadowed state of self-hate. In wanting to escape my reality so desperately, I had ventured into some dark places, losing all respect for men along the way. I came to understand, of course, that it wasn't actually men I had lost respect for. It was myself. Most men are beautiful, vulnerable beings. It had nothing to do with men. It had to do with me. So I apologized to my body for the thoughts and actions associated with those days, too.

Despite the flak that had often been directed at me from particular family members, I also felt awful for the way I had handled my responses. There had been many times when I had replied to attack with attack. In later years, I learned to reply to attack with self-defense, which felt much better. Thankfully, I had then evolved further, where I could respond with neither. I could respond with either silence or with kindness and compassion. Meditation, especially, had tapped my mind into the heart and power of compassion. It was a much better approach than attack, defense, or a need to be right.

Previously I had certainly off-loaded some verbal cruelty in response to the same from others. Although I wasn't attracting those situations anymore, I still needed to forgive myself for what I *had* said.

There were those and so many more apologies to myself. It wasn't the apologies that were the most important, though. It was my ability to *accept* my apology by truly and wholly forgiving myself.

There were plenty of things I would have changed about my past, but I wasn't willing to live with regret. Caring for dying people had blessed me with so many vital lessons about that. I had already spent enough of my life in harsh judgment of myself. While I didn't really feel I had been in that place for some time now, I obviously hadn't reached a place of complete forgiveness yet.

So I stood regularly at the mirror, looking into the depths of my own eyes, usually crying, and learned to forgive myself. I was not only saying sorry. I was learning how to receive and wholeheartedly accept those apologies. I was learning how to love myself enough to forgive.

With a compassionate heart, I reassured myself that it was okay. The past *was* forgiven, and it was time to start moving forward free of harsh self-judgment. I had done my best as the person I was at the time. Now, as the person I had become, I could look back and love that broken person for who she was then. I forgave my actions, my thoughts, and my words. *I forgave myself!*

The liberation I felt from this breakthrough was astounding. It brought a new lightness to my heart. I felt more connected to my child-self, who lived within me: a being once so free and able to allow love to flow without consideration. It was a glimpse of my potential return to joy. Forgiveness was the first turn of the key.

It was time to learn how to embrace happiness—without guilt. A new determination also rose to shatter the upper limits that kept bumping my head every time my life took a step upward.

I no longer cared about time and how long it was going to take. I had a disease and was going to milk it completely for every lesson it offered. Faith in the healing journey and trust in the big picture would give me the strength to keep going, one step at a time.

13

Somewhere along the road, my young, possibly unconscious mind had decided I didn't deserve to be happy. Words spoken to me during my childhood and as a young adult surfaced. My restlessness and sense of adventure had been criticized regularly, accompanied by accusations of me being hopeless and not deserving happiness. It was really just my own interpretation of these words that actually hindered my sense of worth for happiness.

By now I had come to understand no one can have power over us unless we allow him or her to. However, it takes a lot of conscious effort, time, and love to undo the old ways of thinking. When we think we have undone it all, yet another layer goes and reveals itself.

Having a delightful little girl around me discovering the world through eyes of wonder and joy certainly reconnected me with the idea of happiness—and my somewhat damaged concept of it. While I had always considered myself optimistic and fairly resilient, a new yearning was growing. It was a desire to capture happiness through innocence again, to reconnect with unhindered joy.

Before that destination could be reached, it seemed that my healing path had other ideas. Seeing my own little self through my daughter's example, I began to experience anger that surprised the life out of me. It had been deeply suppressed and now insisted on bubbling up. I grew *extremely* angry.

Once, I too had been as sweet, innocent, and loving as my dear little girl. I too had been as deserving of love as she definitely was. Now I witnessed the love my father gave to Elena so freely, and it killed me. Of course, I would not have accepted him being any other way with her. Had he shown her even a glimpse of how he had treated me, I would have removed us from his life entirely.

There was no way her childhood was going to be ruined in the same way I felt mine had been.

Nonetheless, struggles of pain surfaced. Why had I had to live in terror of his rage? Why had I been the brunt of his cruelty? Why did he find it so easy to love Elena when I had been just as beautiful and deserving? I hated him. *I hated him.* And I hated him even more because I always forgave him.

Then we would go to visit, only because he lived with Mum, and I wouldn't hate him *at all.* I would just see a sad, regretful old man who was doing his best to love his daughter through the love he now gave to her child.

There was so much to be healed. A significantly long time had passed since I'd actually received negative treatment from my father or particular siblings. Still, the past had obviously shaped my long-term perception of worth.

Although I would not have called recent relationships with any of my siblings particularly close, I felt no ill will to any of them anymore. We had all moved on to new places within our relationships. When I used to live away, I often felt as if I was missing out on being a part of the big, happy family. Moving back, I discovered that although they saw one another at times, they were all busy getting on with their own lives.

I would always be the black sheep—and that was okay. The idea of socializing around barbecues and alcohol held absolutely no interest for me anyway, and how I chose to spend my time was becoming a growing priority. Being ill was giving me permission to make more conscious choices of what I said yes and no to.

Despite the illness and a gorgeous toddler, visits from siblings to my home were still rare. They were all used to me being the visitor. I had no desire to play that role anymore and was too incapacitated to put the effort in regardless. They did all care. They were just busy being who they were. I cared, too, but not enough to play the old roles I used to. I was busy learning how to love me.

So while I no longer felt I held anyone else responsible for my happiness, I was kind enough to myself to acknowledge I had previously allowed their opinions to affect me. I increasingly didn't see them as people whose opinions I needed anymore. Instead, I was grateful for the connections of our souls' journeys and for the blood bond we would always share. But they were just people—nice people, but just people.

In the meantime, I was a person, too, an amazing one who had overcome much. To heal through the disease, irrespective of everything that had shaped my past, I had to change many old habits.

Giving to others had always been easy for me. There was plenty of love in my heart to give. I always let myself stand last in line when handing out my own love and care. My focus was on me now, with my heart calling me to a bigger life, free of old limits.

Strangely, despite the disabilities in my body continuing to increase, my sense of peace grew. Saying no became easier. So did not making plans. This allowed for more moments of stillness, each revealing a new sense of peace in who I actually was. There were certainly moments of incredible frustration and fragility. But the gradual breakthroughs continued to unfold. Being ill gave me permission to act in new ways. While I didn't want to become dependent on the illness to continue those permissions, more and more I found myself feeling grateful for the situation. Because I was so ill and incapacitated, I was losing my resistance to the disease and surrendering to each day being whatever it would be.

There is power in surrender. It takes courage, but it also brings relief.

14

The more the disease progressed, the further my memory of health retreated. I knew that if I was going to regain my strength, I would need the feeling and hope of health and mobility. Unfortunately, I was too far gone to remember what freedom felt like.

Pain had accompanied me for so long that it was now my reality. I was losing grip of my dreams, unable to even imagine them coming about. Every day they slipped further away, growing smaller and smaller in my vision, until they disappeared out of sight.

There was a certain acceptance to this, though on some days it probably felt more like resignation. The light of hope still burned quietly. It never *fully* diminished, but there were days when I definitely lost sight of it, simply being too blinded in pain and heartache.

I grew in the skill of surrender, finely balancing it on the good days between acceptance and hope. In doing so, I relieved myself of a great deal of resistance, pressure, and expectations.

Surrender allowed me to be present, accepting the moment as it was. It gave me permission to hand it over to God (or whatever we choose to conceive this loving universe to be). I began giving up control, dictating outcomes, or fighting what was. Surrender was a freedom in itself, despite how much courage I often needed to let go. So while my heart was somewhat devastated in having to surrender dreams, it was also more at peace in other ways from acceptance.

Tears could come and go as they needed. Moments of presence and gratitude also broke through, having been given the space to do so. I didn't feel like I *had* to be doing anything. All I had to do was be and take each day as it came. If that meant an afternoon nap with Elena, then great. If it meant saying no to visitors, that was okay. If it meant saying yes to company, sure. The word *should* departed from my life.

While that took the pressure off in all sorts of ways, I did still have to care for Elena. Some days I didn't want to actually get up. The pain of movement was so severe, with the added chronic exhaustion. But the light from my daughter's innocent heart and her complete unconditional love gave me the strength to get up each day.

My mum would take Elena for a few hours regularly when she could, which always helped. One time I called my younger sister and told her clearly that I just wasn't capable of being a mother that day. She delighted in taking Elena off to play with her cousin. But usually my fear of being incapable of keeping Elena drove me to push myself beyond comfortable limits.

There was also my own care that had to be done. Through much research online and personal experience, I was learning an immense amount about diet. By now, I had been living as a vegan for 15 years and as a vegetarian for the 10 years prior. So I had considered myself pretty healthy. Creativity in the kitchen was something I had enjoyed, often pulling together dinner parties for 10 or more people.

With flare-ups of agony arriving regularly, added to the usual ongoing pain in between, I began paying more attention to my diet. Certain foods were definitely not helping. So I embarked upon various dietary paths based on success stories from others with RA.

Gluten was the first to go. I experimented with completely raw, as well as no-sugar, oil-free vegan living, cutting out nightshade vegetables, and on and on. The list of solutions was immense. In desperation I applied myself to each one with renewed commitment. Feeling as though I gave a fair trial to all of them, I kept searching.

Some meals would leave me more inflamed. Others left the inflammation consistent but drained my energy more. Others seemed to suit me okay, but took too long to prepare or left me hungry soon after.

An additional challenge was that I could hardly stand for long enough to prepare food. My hands could not cut through most vegetables anymore either. Every time someone walked in the door to visit, they were greeted with jars to be opened, food to be cut, and things to lift. Eventually my enthusiasm for finding the answer through diet waned, and for a couple of months, I lived on fruit and bowls of gluten-free breakfast cereal with almond milk.

Winter also arrived. The heating in my home was great when it was on, but the house didn't hold the heat. Around three or four in the afternoon, it didn't seem to matter if the house was actually warm or not. The cold shifted into my bones. It was revolting. Not only were the gremlins doing their usual damage on specific joints of their choosing, the bones free of attack throbbed with cold.

When the forecast showed an extra cold snap coming up, I knew I had to get out of there. Being winter and off-season, a fabulous holiday deal presented itself. So off Elena and I went, to warmer climates, about seven hours' drive northeast. The destination was a little coastal village. I'd lived very near to it 15 years earlier. It was also accessible to old friends further north. So for eight wonderful days, I had the support of good mates visiting and the soothing balm of glorious winter sunshine. Our resort was at the beach. Although I couldn't actually walk on the sand, smelling the sea air again was *fantastic*.

Within a day, it became glaringly obvious. I belonged back in this climate. Even if I didn't swim in the ocean every single day, I needed the openness of it. There was also more access to organic food, which was becoming increasingly important to me. Then there was the rain. I needed to be where it was present. I had been raised in severe drought, but had also lived in the tropics, where it poured every day through the wet season. I still *loved* the rain, even after that.

There was also a different consciousness in this area, one that resonated with me. It seemed ludicrous that I had moved back to my home region actually believing I could stay there long-term. Sure, I had wanted my own home, but I would forever be out of place there. That region was dry, farming country. It had magnificent mountains surrounding it, but it hardly ever rained. Recently, I had been feeling like my soul was parched.

There were no regrets in having moved back there. The calling had been so strong that I could not have ignored it. Obviously there was great healing on offer in doing so. Since I had bought my own house and actually lived in my own space, I had a better view of things. It taught me that even in my own house there, I would never actually feel at home. My lifelong yearning for a sense of home in the place of my roots was finally extinguished, and that was perfectly fine.

By the time we headed back south, my decision was clear. We had to move away. I needed to breathe, and life was calling me elsewhere. It was calling me back to the coast and to the rain. It was calling me home.

Naturally there was sadness in telling Mum. She and Elena were so connected, but their bond could never be broken by distance. I, too, would miss the regular sight of Mum. But because I had lived away for so long previously, I knew I would adjust again. Elena would too, wrapped in her mother's love.

My greatest fear was how I would cope without Mum's help. I had grown dependent on her, and she had made herself indispensable. A part of me knew that I needed to ascertain my independence if I was ever going to move forward. Stagnation had suffocated me enough.

I trusted that it was a part of Elena's path to experience this change, too. A happier mother would also make for a much happier childhood. It would certainly be much more fun than the current direction things were heading.

Over the next few months, I had some odd jobs done on the house to prepare it for sale. I had spent a bit of money on doing it up when we moved in. When it sold a month or two later, I had made my money back.

Happily I handed over the keys of a delightfully renovated house to a young couple, full of excitement about their first home.

When Elena and I left, I realized it was the first time I had ever departed from the region with no unsettled feelings at all—no obvious emotional pain, no longing for fulfillment.

I left there in peace.

15

On the last evening of that holiday up the coast, I had come across an article in a magazine in our room. It was an interview of a local naturopath who had worked all over the world but had come home to raise her family. The story was inspiring. It also called me to make an appointment with her.

By the time we had moved from the south, I had traveled up a couple of times to see her. She definitely understood my reluctance and fear in taking the pharmaceutical medications for RA. The confidence I began the journey with to heal the disease was fast slipping away. So it was wonderful to meet someone who not only respected my choices but also felt confident about the possibility of reversing disease.

I had been genuinely surprised that the disease had not already gone into remission or at least shown improvement after all the internal healing I had been going through. There was no way that my body was carrying the emotional pain that it once had been. I had courageously followed whatever guidance I had been intuitively given, both emotionally and physically. So I had felt certain that my health would have caught up to my more peaceful interior by now.

Listening to what the naturopath said, my hope was renewed. I did hit a bit of a wall when she spoke of my need to take a strong fish oil supplement. This was followed by her strong recommendation to actually start eating fish again. After 25 years of vegetarian and vegan life, she may as well have said I needed to bounce around the world backward, balancing on one finger.

Still, chronic pain makes you look at life with more openness. It shakes up all your ideals and throws them to the wind. My walking ability was fast reducing, now restricted to about 100 meters on a good day. I couldn't take Elena to a playground, as I couldn't walk on the grass. Although swimming may have been great for me, getting in and out of a pool was impossible without help. I'd lost confidence to even try it while having to look after Elena's safety in the process.

It was actually the loss of confidence that was increasing most of all. Physical strength gives such self-assurance. It is difficult to realize just how much, until it has been taken away. My weight continued to fall, well past the point of me looking a healthy slim. I looked ragged. I *was* ragged. I was frail, bent over, and broken, wearing a constant look of pain on my face.

I gave in to the suggestion and returned fish to my diet. Although I struggled with it a bit at first, *a lot* actually, my resistance did ease over time. My diet was still predominantly vegan. Our bodies change and evolve. I had to allow my diet to flow with those changes, even if I was still working through the moral side of the new diet.

With more suitable foods and some herbal tinctures, my health improved a little—in that it appeared to slow down the progression of the disease. I hung in there, having been advised that natural remedies take longer than pharmaceutical medications to show their effects. So I kept going one step at a time.

In the meantime, I started to browse online for walking sticks. The assurances that physical balance and strength had silently offered were long gone, but it was not only their absence that robbed my confidence. I was increasingly terrified of falling over and not only being unable to get up but of breaking a bone in the process. Then who would look after Elena? Just to walk down a slight step of a few inches, I had to steady the balance of my frail body on a pole, holding on to it for dear life as my shaky legs dared to move a little bit at a time. As confidence and strength slipped away further each day, fear increased tenfold.

Elena and I were making friends easily in the new location even though I was certainly declining more invitations than accepting them. The thought of any venture was painful and exhausting. I was also weary of the attention the disabilities attracted. But for Elena's sake, I forced myself to be sociable and get us out and about when possible.

From the beginning of my role as a mother I fully embraced the learning as much as I could. I felt incredibly grateful I could work from home. It is a well-documented fact your time is the biggest gift you can give your child. Various teachings on conscious parenting were resonating with me—all in the direction of treating the child as a person, with respect and guidance rather than through control and creating fear.

Elena was allowed to have meltdowns, as toddlers do. They have some pretty big emotions and don't know any other way to release them. I would assure her of my love regardless. Having been too scared to express myself in my own childhood, there was no way I was willing to hinder Elena's spirit. As a result of the choices I tried to make as consciously as possible, or perhaps just because she was who she was, Elena was fast becoming a confident little girl. Her conversation skills were advanced, as were her curiosity and ability to express herself.

Through my continued learning as a mum, I also came to a very clear conclusion about the many benefits of homeschooling when done well. So when she was two years old, we began connecting with other homeschooling families. Her social network grew easily, providing much fun for Elena and positive connections for me. Outings were planned. When the children asked about bees, we visited the bee farm and watched honey being made. If they wanted to know about colors, we encouraged their inquiring minds with experimentation of paints.

There were still old friends in my life from my previous chapter in the area, and positive people increasingly surrounded us. But owing to mounting disabilities, the social side of life was kept to a minimum. I would return from brief outings totally exhausted. Elena had now decided to forgo her daytime naps, which removed that gift from me, too. Life was getting way too hard. Pain was drawn permanently on my face. Bones protruded through increased loss of weight. I would think twice when doing things around the house, being influenced by how I might be able to save myself walking an extra two steps.

With such confined restrictions, life was mostly devoid of physical freedom. Yet it offered a lot of time for sorting through thoughts and observing myself. It was a gift of time for much con-templation, amongst the tears and heartache that still surfaced.

It was a time to look at what I now believed and what I was willing to accept, all in the name of healing and growth.

My thoughts were certainly changing.

At least something was.

16

As I had a reasonable excuse to say no to a lot, it began to shape my new ways of thinking. Being ill was definitely teaching me to be gentle on myself in all areas. The layers I had worked through in self-forgiveness were also freeing me up immensely. This was becoming a skill more easily embraced when needed.

There were days I could have handled things better—as a parent, or in any aspect of my life. But I could forgive myself now, and love myself for whomever I was that day. My heart opened with compassion, as it would for anyone suffering. It was not a failure to get sick. It would only be a failure if I insisted on blocking it all out and not learning from the experience.

Illness was a fabulous teacher. I realized that through it, I was now actually living much of the life I had dreamed of. Without a doubt, being disabled had taught me how. I was working from home in a job I loved. My working hours were minimal. With a laptop computer, I had the freedom to live anywhere.

When the right speaking engagement came along, I accepted it. I said no to others if they were not going to leave me feeling good, either emotionally or physically. I was still not working outside the home very much at all. Physically, I was not yet capable of doing so, but having that excuse also reinforced the new habit of permitting myself to say no. I may have achieved this with full health, but what was different was my ability to say no *without guilt*.

Money also no longer shaped my decisions. I wasn't so cashed up that I didn't have to work. I did. Yet decisions about earning were no longer based around fear of lack with money. The choices were shaped by whether something was going to leave me feeling good or not.

With this new habit of decision making, my faith also increased. I had worked *so* hard to get my message heard and to reach the level of success I was now enjoying. Success to me was not only about being able to make a living from something I loved, but also about having time to enjoy balance and real-life relationships.

To truly love my work, there had to be heart involved and a sense of contribution. As I had created a job into which I could put a heartfelt attitude, in my own eyes I was already a success, regardless of what income was flowing. When I felt as though I was helping others in some way, I felt a sense of connection with the greater whole.

As that feeling of contribution had become ingrained in my career path, I trusted I would be looked after. Day by day, old habits were shifting. Expectations were also rising. My role as a receiver, not just as a giver, was beginning to fit me better. Most times when I was offered help, I accepted it. Each time I did, there was much less resistance than the time before. It actually felt nice to receive. I loved that it gave the other person an opportunity to give, as I had often enjoyed that feeling myself previously.

As well as loving my work, the gratitude and pleasure I experienced in being Elena's mother was overwhelming. I would look at her, so pure and full of delight, and constantly be amazed by the role I was now living. For a couple of decades as an adult, my path was solitary (despite a couple of long-term relationships). Little did I know that this divine little being was just floating nearby all that time, waiting for the right moment to incarnate as my daughter.

On top of that, I was able to stay at home as a mum, being very present for Elena. Two days a week she had delightful care elsewhere, enabling me to remember who I was outside parenthood. Elena loved that time with her friends, and even though I always missed her, it enabled me to write and attend to business.

As there was only the two of us, we had complete freedom to allow our days to unfold as they would. If we wanted to eat out at a café, we did. If we wanted our main meal at home at 3 P.M., no worries. Playtime could go on and on. If I wasn't well enough to visit the whole-foods store, then it waited for another day. The day could be whatever it wanted to be, with room to breathe.

Space was indeed the biggest gift. Increased consciousness about this was a result of being ill. As I didn't know from one day to the next how I would be feeling, it had become essential to leave space in my days. I was learning to not try to fit in too much anymore. The pressure we all unnecessarily learn to put on ourselves was lifted from me. Having space in my days became a new habit, one that was enriching life enormously.

Being stagnant, physically, for so long was certainly a challenge. It had been about two and a half years since I had been able to exercise. Even yoga was too hard. I embraced qigong for some time through a home program. Perhaps if I had discovered that earlier in the diagnosis, I would have been able to stick it out. It was hard to remain inspired, though, when every movement was acutely painful.

After consistently huge efforts in finding a solution, I was becoming tired again. Not only was I exhausted physically; I was tired of trying. The feeling of being well had slipped so far from my memory that it was increasingly difficult to imagine life beyond illness.

What God especially wanted me to learn and master was to allow rather than to strive. Being incapable of striving anyway, allowing was becoming my new habit. Life was much gentler when lived from that state.

My time effectively became more productive. No longer was there unnecessary activity. When I was truly guided to take capable action, I did, but in more productive ways. Our loving universe did the rest.

In its own way, it was actually becoming a wonder-filled way to live. Instead of struggling, I opened more each day to surprise and the infinite creativity of God.

17

By reaching such acceptance and having the permission to go slower, day-to-day life became more manageable. The pain was still there. In fact, it was increasing. But pockets of bliss rose to the surface. Tears of gratitude also sprang up spontaneously. Being present shifted my senses, bringing me alive again.

Something else that was changing was my feeling toward being online. I had been sitting on my backside now for a *long* time, still unable to exercise despite my wishes. As a result, the computer had become an even more significant part of my world.

In many ways, my dreams were kept alive through the Internet. There was a growing yearning to visit New York. Although I had lived in other foreign cities, New York had not yet become a part of my experience. The melting pot of humanity, food, entertainment, chaos, and pace all enticed me. Too much time in stagnation added to that yearning. Of course, the dream of New York also included my ability to walk for endless hours discovering the nooks and crannies of the city. At this stage, I couldn't even wear running shoes. Nor could I walk more than 30 meters at a time. So it was a big dream. Other dreams were also researched and planned online.

Eventually, however, a festering aversion to being online grew until I could no longer ignore it. As work went, the Internet was essential. I also loved the convenience of it, the freedom to live anywhere as a result. The connection I shared with my readers and listeners was very real, too, keeping me on track to continue serving in the ways I did. So much genuine love flowed between us. It was not only from me to them, but from them to me. Great work relationships also existed.

But I was sick of sitting on my bum. It began driving me crazy. So did being online more than absolutely necessary. I hired a virtual assistant to do some of my administrative work. More so, I began to use my online time more efficiently, making a conscious effort to not linger any longer than I had to.

It was not only my physical freedom that I was missing. Through all of the time online and incapacitation, I missed real life. I longed for face-to-face conversations, having the energy for phone conversations instead of text messages, smiling at strangers, being out and about, just general life that didn't involve a computer. Even if I couldn't walk on sand, sitting in the car looking at the ocean was healthier for me than looking at a computer screen.

So I gifted myself with further liberation by reclaiming more time offline. It made a significant difference. Somehow it enabled me to start seeing myself through clearer eyes. When you become so ill over time, it is hard to view your own demise. It is like being in a disempowering relationship, or having a drug or work addiction. Every day you lose a little bit more of yourself until one day you look at yourself in the mirror, puzzled. *Who are you?* you wonder. *Where have I gone?*

Despite following the natural therapy advice strictly, my health continued to deteriorate. I was deliberately wearing clothes that hid my protruding shoulder bones and rib cage. There were only a few items I could get in and out of anyway. After I would dress little Elena with my hands screaming in pain, she would help me get dressed or pull clothes off over my head. This divine little being had definitely chosen to learn empathy as a part of her soul's journey. She still had plenty of little girl time, but I hated my increasing dependence on her. I hadn't had a baby so I could have a caregiver.

Around this time, I was introduced to a local doctor. He practiced conventional medicine, but also acupuncture and Ayurvedic medicine. Even though he dealt with pharmaceutical companies, he also spoke my language. He was very respectful of my efforts and choices thus far, and in his quiet, non-threatening manner, he convinced me to seek further help.

I made an appointment with the rheumatologist he recommended. There was a three-month waiting list. Instead of being disappointed, I was grateful. A part of me still hoped for a miracle to avoid going down that road. So I hung on as best I could.

What this time ended up giving me instead of hope was further acceptance. Rather than feeling regret for not having sought this option from the start, I felt gratitude. There had been incredible and valuable learning along the way, wisdom I could never have gained through wellness. I definitely needed help with my physical health now, but my emotional wellbeing was the strongest it had ever been. My spiritual health had also evolved enormously.

It was interesting to realize just how much I had previously expected of myself. I was a solo mum and had raised a baby through all of this. She was now a busy little girl. Yet some days I could hardly lift a teacup. Standing for more than two minutes was unbearable, and still I had continued to rally on, determined to control the healing path and the outcome.

Surrendering was teaching me the best kind of authentic freedom. Eventually I came to the conclusion that just because I could do it tough, didn't mean I had to. The pain had become too severe to go on further anyway. A wheelchair would be the next purchase if I continued.

I decided even if every single potential side effect from the new drugs were to surface in me, it would be still worth it if it gave me just one day off from the pain. That's how desperate I had become for positive change. I was in a *terrible* way—hunched over, wincing with every step, scared of any further movement. Those three months of waiting for the appointment were witnessing the largest demise in my abilities yet.

Instead of being fearful, I became unbelievably peaceful. It was the truest sense of surrender I had experienced. It was out of my hands. I had reached a turning point, with the willingness to let it go in a direction I had resisted. Recognizing how perfect the journey had been so far, for the benefit of my soul's journey and the wisdom it had already gifted me with, I found myself smiling in a new way. Whatever lay ahead would all be okay. If I could continue to look for the blessings, I would continue to find them.

Despite attempts by increasingly raging pain to leave lasting memories, I started to become deliriously happy. Something in me was shifting well past peace. It was not enough anymore. Joy was the destination now calling. My body was in agony, aching to intense new levels. Yet laughter was returning to my life. Acceptance became my greatest freedom.

Admitting to myself that I actually *wanted* an easy life was also liberating. As I had not chosen to stay in the corporate world and had drifted a lot in previous years, I had been labeled as lazy by some of my family. Perhaps they were jealous of my courage and freedom, although I didn't know that back then as a young adult. Instead, I had been doing my penance ever since, attracting one hardship after another to justify the balance. How could I have a great life, simply a great life, without some form of hardship? Oh, the way the mind weaves!

Now I could speak it out loud. Instead of feeling ashamed, guilty, or concerned by others' opinions, it felt wonderful to admit it. I wanted an easy life. It was okay to want and *have* an easy life. *It was okay!*

It didn't mean I denied my roles as a parent, artist, businesswoman, or whatever the situation called for. They were all a part of it. But how many things I overcame were irrelevant if I didn't create a different life beyond them. Repeating the same patterns would not have been an achievement. They would have been warning signs.

There had to come a time when I reached the threshold of what I was willing to endure. RA opened my eyes to that. If I continued to accept more and more hardship, then life would keep giving me what I expected.

So, no more! I wanted an easy life, and I could sing it from the rooftops. I didn't express or feel it in a defensive way or in defiance to anyone either. I felt it with pure joy and love of myself. This simple sentence was one of the most wonderful insights I'd ever allowed myself to feel. It was setting me free. It was okay to want and have an easy life.

So instead of walking into the rheumatologist's office full of fear and a sense of failure at the end of those three months, I felt delighted to embrace whatever lay ahead. If I could have skipped in there, I would have. I hobbled instead, but I hobbled happily.

18

With little Elena in tow, content to play on the floor with her blocks, I sat on the chair in the specialist's office. Telling my story was quite unnecessary. My body could talk for itself. I saw the instant recognition in his eyes of where I was. Still, he listened with patience and respect.

He was a kind man and very gentle as he felt my swollen hands. If I had any energy for romance in my life, I could have almost fancied him in a doctor-patient sort of way. I liked his manner a lot and was relieved I had waited to see him specifically.

It felt like the printer was working overtime as it produced the list of potential side effects for the medications he spoke of. Expressing my fears, he was reassuring in an experienced, knowledgeable way. I was too far gone anyway. It was time to try them. We would meet in another month, after I'd had more blood tests. The medications could do lifelong damage to other organs, so blood tests would be a regular thing in order to monitor the whole picture.

It would take about six weeks for the first medication to kick in properly. Then after three months, we would add another one to the cocktail. Still, I felt hopeful.

Over the next month I waited in anticipation for improvement. Pain was constant, but there had been no enormous flare-ups during that time. The raging disabling monster seemed to be settling. I noticed, too, that my jeans were feeling a little tight.

As I had moved house so regularly before because of a love of relocating and house-sitting opportunities, I was great at culling my belongings. It drove me a little crazy to have anything in my home that was not useful or being worn regularly.

As a result, I had given away all my regular-size clothing over the previous couple of years since they were all too big for me.

Now all I owned were small clothes and not many of those. Most styles were too hard to get in and out of. Shopping and trying on clothes had been such a burden that I'd just stuck with my absolute basics. But now I was in strife. Weight was returning and I had nothing to wear. Off to the charity shop I went. It seemed ridiculous to buy anything new when I had no idea what my body would do over the coming months.

What it did end up doing was return 15 kilograms to my weight within three months. Fifteen! My diet had remained as before. The only real changes were the medications and the amount of energy my poor body had been using to deal with the level of intense and constant pain. As the agony shifted to more tolerable levels, my body now piled on more than I even wanted. Weight wasn't my current priority, though.

Comfort and increasing abilities were much more important. Day by day, month by month, subtle improvements continued. I could open a particularly difficult door with more ease. The length of time I could stand increased a little. The frown of pain on my brow became more occasional. And my attention span increased gradually.

With every visit back to the rheumatologist, we shared delight in the changes. On seeing my blood tests after the first month, he told me that for someone as sick as I was, I was the healthiest person he'd seen. So basically, keep doing what I was doing, but do his recommendations as well.

Some side effects did surface. Had I not been to the agonizing places I'd already been with the disease, I might have been more concerned. But not only can some other effects from RA actually kill you; so can pain itself. It takes an enormous toll on the body. When I weighed it all up, I had to accept and hope that the risks and current side effects were less damaging than the path I had been walking. Plus, if I wanted to remain living independently without a wheelchair and full-time caregiver, this was my best choice.

Some days when flare-ups did happen, feeling like I was slipping backward almost broke my heart. But rather than see it as a catastrophe, I would try to turn it around. The flare-ups were less frequent. I was growing stronger. While pain was always there in some capacity, it was not so distracting. Also, as I had already learned, it was perfectly okay to take days off from plans and just be. This would remain a part of the ride, it seemed. Now and then, regardless of improvement, there were days when I just had to let go.

The best thing the improvements did was reconnect me with memories of who I used to be. I had been a country girl, once strong and healthy. I had never had a naturally slim build, but I had been strong and I liked that. The memory of strength pulled me forward.

Many restrictions remained, but not all. When I was learning to play the guitar several years earlier, I came to understand how the fingers remembered where to go without the brain consciously directing them every step of the way. So I considered muscle memory in relation to my strength.

Even if I was blessed with spontaneous remission, something I did still hold a glimmer of hope for, my muscles had been dormant for nearly three years. They needed waking up. They needed to remember how to be strong again. If I was ever going to regain the physical freedom I was daring to imagine, it was up to me to begin my own rehabilitation.

Ever so slowly I tried to reintroduce a little yoga back into my life. There were many postures that were still impossible, mostly any putting pressure on my wrists. That didn't mean there were not some I *could* do. So I began, for just a few minutes a day. I couldn't believe my once-flexible body could be so rigid, but it was never going to become flexible in any capacity again without effort.

One day while at playgroup with Elena, I was speaking with one of my mum friends. She was sitting on the floor playing with her new babe. I commented on how I missed being able to do that. Even with improvements, I was scared to try it. If I managed to sit on the floor and could not get up, what would I do? There was only me and Elena at home. She was a strong little thing, for sure, but not that strong!

My friend suggested I try it there, where she and another mother could help me up if needed. Despite agreeing, I was still terrified. My backside made it almost to the floor as I lowered myself against the side of a sofa, but I had to fall the last few inches. Having no strength in my hands or wrists, I tried to maneuver myself to rise. The two women instructed me on the best way to do it. My toes would not take pressure on standing, so I used my elbows, pushing up onto the nearby sofa, using any strength available. I am sure my tongue was out whilst deep concentration unfolded.

Then I did it. I stood up. All the way from the floor! If I could have jumped in the air to celebrate, I would have. With a huge smile, I raised my arms up in a gesture of achievement. Then I promptly burst into tears.

Years of heartache, frustration, and anguish surged out of me. My friend's loving smile, as her babe now nursed on her breast, was just what I needed. It nurtured me through the release. When the tears finally eased, I put myself back on the floor and rose again. This was repeated a few times.

The freedom of this movement, one most of us take for granted on a daily basis, was life changing. It not only meant I could sit on the floor and play with my little girl at her level, it meant a bath may even be a possibility. If there was something I could hold in order to stand, sitting on the earth might also happen again. I longed to reconnect with nature—to just sit on grass or a rock. This achievement not only gave me increased possibilities; it offered renewed confidence. I had indeed turned a corner. A new me was being born.

19

Who is to say what might have happened if I had gone onto medication straight away? We all have our own life lessons to learn, our own journey to travel. Without reaching such a low place, I would never have become who I had.

Many people immediately look for a science-based solution through pharmaceutical medications. Others go straight to natural-based therapies. Some do a blend of both. Another selection of people starts at one and goes to the other. Although the symptoms of disease are similar, every person's travels through their healing are individual. Through every physical challenge, an invitation for further spiritual growth awaits. While some people don't actually cure their disease or it may even be the reason their lives comes to closure, it can still be a healing journey.

Ideally the reversal or cure of disease can occur. I certainly had not lost hope for such. Regardless, my focus was now on building strength and what I *could* do, not on what my restrictions were. It was okay not to deny those. They did exist, but the more my acceptance grew, the less effect they had on my life.

I had to follow my own guidance. There were obviously things I had to learn through RA. There still were. The ride was not over. Although there are many wonderful teachers out there, alternative and otherwise, nothing will beat the wisdom from our own intuitive guidance. And from this perspective I continued to move forward one moment at a time.

There were occasions in the past when I had wondered why I had been guided toward a particular diet or therapy that had not turned out to be the answer for curing the disease. But with the lessons offered, I now saw that every step along the way gently revealed another layer of insights. It educated me on very important matters, including diet and self-care. It brought me into a much closer and more loving relationship with my body. It allowed me to grow at a pace I could manage. I was being taught how to love me.

Just as there is a limit to how much pain we can tolerate, there is one on how much happiness we can allow. As each layer of healing revealed itself, I could adjust gradually to that inner growth, rather than be so overwhelmed I couldn't handle it. There was a reason I learned one step at a time—so I could handle the pace and grow into my new self.

Through the continued practice of surrender and the associated acceptance that grew from it, my focus was no longer on overcoming the disease. The desire to grow strong again was what continued to pull me forward. As it did, I was able to view strength from a whole new angle. Previously, I had not only been very strong physically; I had also been strong emotionally. Life had already sent enough learning my way to ensure as such. Now it was a different strength that I was learning.

My body and heart were in unison as a more wholesome strength revealed itself. Physically, the rebuilding of strength had to be done gently. As I could finally get myself in and out of a swimming pool independently, I added an occasional swim to my time. Much of this was in play with Elena. While I jumped around the pool with her in my arms, my legs were working underneath, growing stronger with each session as muscle memory awakened. Occasional lap-swimming opportunities also came along. It was just wonderful to be in the water.

As I could not rebuild my strength with pressure, I did so lovingly and gratefully. I then realized something about my emotional strength: it had always come from a place of necessity and self-protection. There was a defensive element to it in the sense that I *had* to be strong. Yet through the past three years, I had found strength through surrender and vulnerability. The inner strength that had resulted from that and continued to grow was one based on kindness and gentleness.

There was no being strong because I had to be. I didn't have to be every minute. I could be as vulnerable as I liked and still exist in a blanket of inner strength. It was a wholesome power, gentle. It was *true* strength. My body and emotions were working together. They always had been, but my awareness of this symbiosis increased significantly. They were teaching each other with love.

As I became a little more active, the world began to beckon. So I added another new activity, small sunset walks with Elena. We followed the driveway down the hill, over the little creek, marveled at the sights and sounds of the rainforest on either side, and collected leaves and treasures from nature. Since I could bend a little lower, I could also find new hiding spots at home. Small achievements were enormous gifts.

Being able to lift my little girl up was a dream come true. No longer was I confined to sitting for hugs. My hands weren't strong enough, but while standing, I could now scoop her up with my arm, where she climbed the rest of the way, gripping me with her legs and arms. She was like a monkey. Tears filled my eyes as I held her closely.

The first bath I had on the road to recovery happened at Mum's place. In order to have the confidence to try, I needed a backup plan to get out—in this case Mum assisting me if need be. On a visit back south, I slid into the bath, free of intense fear. Elena hopped in with me for a while, too. It was a very special moment.

When the time came to get out, Mum and my little girl cheered me on from the sidelines as I found a way to rise on my own, depending on my elbows. I did it. Another freedom was returned. If I could bathe and swim independently, I would be okay. Something quiet and knowing within assured me I was actually going to be more than okay.

20

When I was a young teenager, my father won some money in the lotto. It wasn't such a huge amount that our physical lives were altered drastically. What it did was enable my parents to purchase the farm we were renting at the time and carry us through the years of severe drought that followed. So it was indeed a blessing to a struggling family.

As we were horse riders and sometimes attended competitions, it was vital to have a reliable vehicle to pull the horse trailer. My parents had purchased a new car, practical and strong enough for the load it had to pull but far too posh for my liking. As a young teenager, I was hugely embarrassed by it. If Mum had to pick me up from school, I would ask her to park down the street so none of my friends would see the car. It took me months before I even mentioned to my close friends that my family had won the money. I was obviously already shaped by upper-limit restrictions. Prior to the win, I had often worried about how Mum and Dad would feed us all.

Life carried on for the family, but things had changed in my father's mind. Winning the lotto was a reality, not just a fantasy. He knew it could be done. So from that time onward, he steadfastly believed he would win it again. He played weekly, not obsessively when it came to what he spent, but doing his numbers became a big part of his life.

As well as being a guitarist, radio announcer, and farmer, he was an accountant. He loved numbers. Each week, he would note which ones came up. On a self-ruled graph, he would note which numbers hadn't come up for ages. He would then begin playing those. When I told him years later you could look those facts up online, it didn't matter. No, he had his system and would not budge from doing it his way each week. No one dared disturb him during this precious time. He swore that number 26 would come up soon, as it hadn't been drawn for ages.

When I was pregnant and living back under his and Mum's roof, there was a regular ad on the TV. It showed a father presenting his daughter with a check to pay off her mortgage. The tagline of the ad for the lottery company was, "Wouldn't it be nice?" Whenever that was on, Dad would tell me he was going to buy me a house one day. I'd just smile and not believe a word of it. I was too determined to buy my own house. A wounded part of me also didn't want to give him the pleasure of doing it, even though a more evolved part of me would have gratefully accepted it.

It was just another of Dad's ways to let me know he cared after all the years of hurt. My relationship with him had certainly been one of my biggest teachers. The period of suicidal depression, followed by the journey with disease, were definitely incredible teachers, too. In fact, they were the healing chapters I needed, for the lessons ingrained from my earlier life. Wounds connected with my father had shaped too much of that.

Now he was doing his best to make amends, and I was doing my best to receive his kinder intentions. Through his own earlier examples, my father had taught me everything I didn't want to be. I silently thanked him for that. I'd also had to find my own happiness over the decades, irrespective of having my father's love and approval.

As much as he tried to create a present relationship, I had reached a place somewhat free of its need. Even if he gave positive feedback—something new for him—it was a little like water off a duck's back. My happiness no longer depended on his opinion or approval.

I did try to view our relationship as the teacher it was in my life and as an avenue to continue growing in compassion. He was an old man trying to make amends. His desire to buy me a house by winning the lottery again was heartfelt. I didn't need him to buy me one. I knew I would find a way myself, which I had, in their village.

When Elena and I moved away from the area later, my father always insisted on accompanying my mother to visit us. We would all meet in a halfway town—about a three-and-a-half-hour drive for us all. Dad's health was deteriorating, so we would book a comfortable apartment for the night to enable rest before the return trip. He always went to bed especially early, but at least he was there. He even began taking an interest in my work. Back at their home, he was unable to put my first book down, staying up until three in the morning to finish reading it. Although he said nothing to me, he apparently told all of his friends about it and recommended they buy it. Bless him.

There was a lot going on with his health, a lot going wrong. There was no terminally diagnosed disease, but there was so much else starting to fail that his quality of life had diminished further each time I saw him. Eventually the overnight trips became too much for him. Yet he still insisted on coming, with the drive becoming a day trip instead. We would meet in a park, where Elena could play and burn off some of her cooped-up toddler energy.

It came to the point where he couldn't even get out of the car except to use his walking frame to get to the toilet. He'd then return to the car and sit there watching us three girls catching up on the playground. At some point, I would leave Mum and Elena in the park and go to him. We'd sit in the car and chat, him asking me about my work and my health. I'd fill him in on it all. When I asked about his health, he would shrug with a philosophical comment about just getting through each day as best he could.

The whole of the east coast of Australia is separated by a magnificent mountain range, appropriately called the Great Dividing Range. As you drive from east to west, the lush green coastal land gives way to arid golden plains. No matter where you're traveling across the range, there comes a time to traverse the midpoint of bushland and winding roads before your descent to the other side.

It was at such a time whilst driving to collect Elena from a weekend with her grandparents that I felt it would be the last time I would be seeing my father. As I covered familiar roads, steep climbs, and hairpin turns, tears flowed freely. I needed Dad to know all was forgiven, that I loved him despite my aloofness at times.

While we sat in the car that day, I held his hand. We chatted on the usual subjects, but there was a closeness and silent understanding between us. There was no need for me to bring it up and cause him pain, to even say things were forgiven. He had enough regrets. That was obvious. So with gentle affection and comfortable silence, we sat holding hands, watching Mum and Elena play in the park.

When they came over, we all squashed into the car and took a selfie on my phone. I hugged my dad good-bye that day, knowing in my heart he could die peacefully with regard to our relationship. There was an unspoken understanding exchanged with our eyes in parting. There was love.

He was still a hard man to many, but I could see through his fear. There was a delicate soul in there, one who'd grown up in a time when men were expected to suppress their sensitivity. In the end, his vulnerability opened the door to his heart and let me in. My own vulnerability finally let him back in, too. He was forgiven. He was loved.

Another month or so passed where further complications arose with his health. Still he played his numbers each week. One spring day, he was sent to the hospital after his legs had swollen to the size of bowling balls. His tender heart was collapsing. It was time to rest now.

Sadly for Dad, number 26 didn't come up again before he died peacefully in his sleep the following night. He was out of pain, though. It was his time.

21

Gratitude and peace were what I experienced most in adjusting to life without my father being physically present. I had grieved for his love for most of my life. When I had reached a place in myself where I no longer needed it, I received it. Life once again reminded me of the nature of surrender. When we lose the attachment to an outcome, we actually open the flow to what our heart is yearning.

So rather than experience a sense of loss, I felt gratefulness. My final memory of him was a tender, beautiful one. We had been blessed with the time to find genuine peace in our relationship, bringing the depth of our love to a very special place. I found myself smiling softly much more than crying.

Of course, there *were* tears too. It was not an all-consuming grief. It was a gentle adjustment to life without my dad. When the first Christmas without him arrived, I definitely missed hearing his deep voice wishing me happy Christmas. So I sent him love through a teary smile. That night he visited my dream.

It was at a social club. Dad didn't venture out much in the end, but he loved going to the local club for lunch with Mum on special occasions. In the dream, he was sitting at a table. There were other people about. I asked myself whether it was real, whether Dad was still alive or not. Then I saw an ashtray full of cigarette butts in front of him. (He had been a very heavy smoker but had quit the habit two decades earlier.) Once I saw the ashtray, I realized the scenario wasn't real, as you can't smoke in Australian clubs anymore. I knew he was in a different place, that it was a dream. I went over and said hello. He smiled and asked if I was doing okay. I smiled and told him that I was.

I mentioned I had to go the hospital for some tests. He was easily accepting, saying, "No worries, Love. I was just checking that you're doing okay." I thanked him, said good-bye with a smile, and walked away through a door into a hospital room. A doctor came in stating that they'd made a mistake. Everything was fine and they didn't need to do any tests. So I left, feeling grateful. If I hadn't been called to the hospital for the tests, I would not have walked through the club and seen Dad.

When I woke in the morning, a loving feeling lingered. Dad had felt my sadness and love on Christmas morning and dropped in that night to let me know he was okay and still looking out for me. I felt very blessed.

Love transcends all realities. Love is love, after all. When I used to work caring for terminally ill people, I'd often been reminded of this. The loving energy in the room of a dying person sometimes felt so palpable that I could almost reach out and touch it. There were also patients who smiled joyfully just prior to their final breath. Only love could do that. Dad and I were still connected. He had dropped in to say hello, just to connect with and reassure me. Our relationship could still continue. It was an exchange of the heart. He felt my love and sent some of his back.

My relationship with Dad had been such a painful one for us both. If we had not cared, though, it would never have hurt. Feeling our connection continuing past the death of his body made all the learning worth it. It showed me it truly is only ever about love.

My heart was continually expanding, helping me have greater empathy, understanding, and kindness. Dad's passing reminded me yet again that it truly can be a magnificent journey. Every lesson offered was about love. If I was going to enjoy increasing peace and flow, including health, abundance, and happiness, then I needed to keep peeling back the layers around my heart. With courage, I continued on.

My trust in the big picture helped me keep looking for the beauty in life and finding it. It reinforced that it was okay to care for me, too. Dreaming of a better life and working toward that was actually natural and perfectly fine.

What wasn't natural and perfectly fine was to do it with ridiculous pressure. So it was becoming a more joyful process by the day as I increasingly removed pressure, trusted in divine timing, and, above all, moved forward with love in my heart.

It was my job to learn to love myself, to expose my heart and continue honoring my dreams. The more connected I became to my own heart's voice, the more it would steer me to serve others. It could do so in a way that would empower me too, though, rather than it being an unbalanced exchange of giving to others, followed by exhaustion and burnout, both physically and emotionally.

I felt blessed to be experiencing these lessons in the ways I was. Life wanted me to see dreams realized. I would not have been given the ability to imagine them otherwise. Aspiration was my heart's voice spoken in one of its clearest tones. My dreams might be manifesting in completely different images than originally considered, but those feelings I had longed for were being answered. It simply took courage to let them flow. I continued to find it through the path of self-care, one step at a time.

The months following my father's departure from physical life brought a rush of insights and courage. Even though Dad was nothing but supportive in the later years, I experienced a new sense of freedom in myself.

The ceiling on my upper limits was opening to increasing light day by day. The more I learned to treat myself kindly, the more life taught me I didn't have to strive so hard. I had to take action when guided. In times in between, my job was simply to continue developing my love for myself so I could become a more opened vessel for things to flow through.

22

The return of health and strength was my heart's biggest longing. The other major dream manifesting was to find our home. It wasn't just a house I was looking for. It was *home*.

For 27 years, I had not lived in any one region for more than two years at a time, often much less. The itch for adventure and discovery, along with my inner restlessness, saw me relocating almost as soon as I started to feel settled. Belongings weighed me down and were often off-loaded, with me picking up replacement furniture and the like when needed. I became a master manifester! So many things flowed to me without effort.

On top of my relocations, there were also some years of house-sitting thrown in. I would move on, anywhere from two weeks to six months at a time. It also meant I lived in some pretty amazing homes. Although those experiences were indeed fabulous in many ways, eventually exhaustion of that lifestyle did arrive.

After buying the house in my parents' village, I realized how much I enjoyed being a home owner. Even though I had a relationship with the bank because of the mortgage, it was still mine. There was no landlord. There were also no rules or restrictions on my creative expression. I loved that feeling. Being a mother and much more settled in myself, as well as being disabled and frail, thoughts of settling into one home for a very long time grew more and more enticing.

Once I made the decision to relocate to the warmer weather, I had put my house on the market. In the meantime, I was searching for something to buy. As the housing markets were vastly different in the two regions, a four-bedroom home with a large yard and established trees in the old region equated to a two-bedroom apartment in the new one.

Privacy in my home environment was paramount for my enjoyment and wellbeing. It wasn't as if I were having wild parties or doing anything that exciting. Growing up on the farm with neighbors so far away planted some essential factors in me. I needed to live where no one could see me coming and going within my home and yard, and where no one could hear me laughing, crying, singing, or talking. I desired complete privacy and unrestricted freedom to be me in whatever mood struck. However, I also wanted accessibility. Having lived in so many places and situations, I'd come to know privacy without isolation would work for me long-term.

Five years earlier I could not even afford to feed myself. There were also millions of members of our human family who did not have food or a home. Sometimes 10 people lived in one room. So I knew there were things to be grateful for, just to be able to buy *at all*. In my heart, though, I really did want *the* home, not just *any* home. Regardless, logic tried to get in the way, insisting I should just buy something, anything.

After a house-hunting trip up north prior to moving there, I had put in an offer on an apartment. It had a glimpse of the river, so I hoped it would assist my balance and wellbeing. There were very steep steps down to the laundry and garage. My incredibly tender and painful feet were begging me not to buy it. Still I proceeded, reasoning in a conversation with God that if it was not meant to be, then please stop it from happening.

The pest and building inspections were ordered and paid for. I began packing up my old house. The bank was contacted with the details of the new place. Everything was flowing and then the phone call arrived. It was the building inspector telling me to keep well clear of the place. Even though the pest report showed no current signs of termites, the building report spoke of extensive damage in the framework, flooring, and walls. He said unless I wanted to live in it forever, I definitely shouldn't buy it as I would never be able to sell without *major* work being done first. My feet breathed immediate relief.

So I smiled and thanked God for intervening. It was too late to start searching for another place before I moved, so the pressure to buy was off. If I had to rent for a while, no worries, I would. After three of my rental applications were refused amongst the dozens of other people applying for the same properties, I asked for clearer guidance. On to a bed-and-breakfast site I went.

A little furnished cottage in the rainforest was available, only about one kilometer from where I had lived in the region years prior. In a brief e-mail to the owner, I shared we were looking for something for either two weeks or two months. If I found a place to rent, it would be two weeks. If I found a place to buy, it would be two months for the legalities to go through. The owner was fine with that. In fact, she was delighted. She had just listed the property for the first time ever, only a few hours before my e-mail arrived.

Once again, before moving I gave away many of my belongings, particularly furniture, though I kept the basics this time as we would need them soon enough. In the meantime everything remaining went onto a truck and straight into a storage shed.

We arrived to a warm, friendly welcome in our new and temporary home. Weekly cleaning was also included, which was wonderful. I was still too frail to do most things, including changing the sheets on the bed. Even when rolling over in the night, I depended on my teeth to pull the sheets back over me. My hands were in too much pain, with fingers that couldn't grip and wrists not strong enough to pull sheets up, let alone fit sheets on a bed or lift a mattress. In all, it was a blessing to find the place when I did.

While my first logical priority might have been to find a rental, it was actually the homes for sale I gave my attention to. My heart felt most peaceful with the idea of finding our own home once and for all.

Whenever I had looked online at real estate, something I'd enjoyed ever since the Internet was born, I was never put off by price. After all, what dream of your castle ever comes with a price tag or a mortgage?

Now I was looking at homes I *could* afford, which were apartments or small townhouses. I did that during practical times. Later, when I would wind down from the day, my search returned to the kind of home I *really* wanted, with no thoughts to price. It was in such a leisurely moment that one particular home stood out to me. My heart quickened when I clicked on it and read more. Something felt right. It didn't matter that the price tag was actually 10 times the price of the little apartment I had tried to buy. Seriously, *10 times* the price. No. No point for logic here. The decision was made then and there. Go and inspect the place. After all, what harm could it do?

I don't know how long it took me to fall asleep that night. It was a long time. With excitement in my heart, I rang the agent first thing the next morning, scheduling an inspection for later that day. Dare I think I could actually own a home like this? Dare I think I could actually break through my upper limits and make this happen? Dare I think? Heck, yes!

So I drove to the inspection with little Elena alongside me. For decades I had been sending out my desires regarding a home and what it would be through my emotions and feelings, both conscious and unconscious. Could this really be the representation of those culminated thoughts?

As we climbed out of the car, a kookaburra laughed from the distance. A magpie garbled in her own delightful song from a tree on the property. Elena ran on ahead. Apparently, she was already home.

23

A simple mud-brick home in the bush was what I had always imagined I would end up in. Yet there were contradictory thoughts about not wanting to be so isolated anymore. Being accessible was not only a strong desire for convenience to services; it was also about being in an easy location for friends to visit. I was done with being the eternal visitor. Still, a mud-brick home had been hanging around for so long that I had never imagined falling in love with something modern-looking, let alone in a suburban cul-de-sac. Yet here I was, about to do just that.

As I walked down the driveway toward the home, a fountain bubbled in the garden. A quiet smile rose from nowhere during those final steps whilst approaching the front door. The moment I entered the spacious, light-filled home, my mind came alive with relief, clearly stating, *I can breathe here*. In all the homes I had lived in, looked after, or visited, I had *never* felt like that. I could breathe. I could truly breathe there.

Besides privacy and accessibility, another essential in my dream home was that the kitchen be in the heart of it. It doesn't matter where people build a kitchen. It still ends up being the busiest and most congregated part of most homes. So why not have the home revolve around the kitchen? Of course, in this particular home, the kitchen was indeed at the very heart of it all.

The view was spectacular, overlooking the swimming pool, then out over the river below, across cane fields, beyond a small town, and on to the glorious Pacific Ocean in the distance. I breathed it all in, feeling the freedom and space to be me. The home reminded me a little of the old farmhouse I grew up in. That one had been as spacious and was similarly on a hill with a big sky view to embrace.

It was not the home I had always imagined, yet it was the dream I had longed for. The feeling I experienced as I walked through, greeting each room as if we had already met long ago, was one of peace and homecoming. Sure, there would be changes I would make to truly call it home. The walls needed more color, as did the furnishings. I told myself the search was over.

All of those years of defining my perfect home were revealed in this one completely unexpected residence. Random thoughts I had experienced had been noted. Feelings I longed for were heard. So many finer details of other characteristics I would have liked in a home but had not considered essential, were there.

My emotions, defined over decades of moving, had all been shaped into a dream, a longing for home. Never did I think that all of those finer details would carry so much significance either. Yet every wish was indeed heard, every longing noted. Now I stood witness to what I had created through the desires of my heart.

Elena picked up a fluffy toy from one of the bedrooms and carried it throughout the rest of the home. Her sense of belonging only added to my excitement, as each room and the garden greeted us with familiarity. She was happy to return the toy at the end of the visit because she was peaceful. We both were. Holding hands, we said good-bye to the agent and walked out the driveway with hope in our hearts.

How could I make this happen? I trusted in the world my dreamer lived within, but if there was a way to assist this happening, I needed to know—and preferably now! With faith and heartfelt sincerity, I prayed for guidance on how I could make this dream become a reality.

The search for other properties was off. There was no point wasting time on false directions. Our home was waiting. I just had to find a way. Really, though, it was not even about finding a solution. Life would provide that clearly enough when the time was right. My job was to grow into the dream, to prepare my readiness.

With confidence, I let our landlord know that we would like to stay on until I could make this dream happen. It suited her perfectly to have ongoing suitable tenants. As we settled more into the rented home with the knowledge it would be for a while longer now, my thoughts were always in the other place.

Any brief moments of leisure online were spent browsing shades of paint, artists' websites for wall hangings, food deliveries, pool maintenance people, and the works. Every search had a purpose. Plans were indeed afoot.

The kitchen came alive with delicious meals cooking and fun-filled times. Hours were spent soaking in baths. Clothes were hung in the walk-in wardrobe. Conversations and laughter unfolded at the dining table. Meditating was done in a perfect setting. Playing in the pool with Elena for hours left me feeling joyfully exhausted. The gym converted into an activity room for Elena and her home-school friends. The tennis court disappeared, transforming into a combined sacred garden and adventure playground. Every day I lived there, in my mind and emotions.

While feeling my way into this dream, plenty of fears also surfaced. I would need help with the maintenance. Some days I could still hardly grip a toothbrush or squeeze the paste out. (My elbows became good at that.) I would definitely require help with the lawns and pool. There was also the embarrassment and unwanted attention of owning the best house on the street. I cringed at inviting certain people there, seeing myself talking down my good fortune or self-worth. Fear after fear surfaced.

Living unnoticed seemed to be a part of my longing, yet life continued to challenge me in its ever so loving and gentle way. Even with my career, I had dealt with fears of being known. They were once enormous until I realized that life really did love me and anything that it was guiding me to do was for the benefit of my inner growth and, hence, my potential happiness. In the big picture, not only had I grown positively from becoming more open; others also benefited through my example of courage. Now another lesson about wanting to be unnoticed seemed to be underway. Why did I have to fall in love with *that* house?

Lovingly I worked my way through every layer of fear. Beneath it all, I believed in the perfection of every day and knew my soul's journey was unfolding in the best way. In my humanness, I continued to grow in compassion for myself while developing more courage. I was also finally able to let myself sit back and reflect on my accomplishments so far, feeling proud instead of talking or thinking them down.

Months rolled by and still we lived as tenants paying rent. The home remained for sale. The price was reduced considerably. An enormous advertising campaign surfaced. The date for auction was set. It came and went, the auction canceled at the last moment. Alone and forlorn the house sat. The owners moved on elsewhere. It was waiting patiently for me. We had met. It was loyal. I just had to bring myself to a place of worth and comfort, in owning and living in such a beautiful home.

Feeling my way forward, I continued to heal more layers. My health and the journey it provided in unison helped delicately chip away more fears. It was a gentle evolution and one I couldn't rush as much as I sometimes wanted to. Deep down, I knew that I probably wasn't quite well enough to enjoy the house properly yet. My walking was so limited it would be hard work living in a bigger home. When every step brought such intense pain, it was easier to take fewer steps by living in a small house.

Questions started to surface within as I challenged some old fears. What was so wrong with enjoying abundance? What was so wrong in admitting that I deserved it? I *did* deserve it! A more evolved part of me knew that comfortably. I had walked my life bravely, always finding the courage to honor my calling, wherever it directed, irrespective of ridicule and fear. I was a good and kind person. Why shouldn't I be living somewhere that was perfect for me?

Courage is always rewarded. Life had proven that to me already through many past experiences. It was trying to do so again by introducing me and the house to each other. It was only through stretching myself that I would be able to reach the sky, or in this case, live in the sky, since the house was on a big hill.

Little by little, I dealt with new layers of recurring fears, trusting that somehow we would be home soon enough. Feeling my way forward, upper limits were revealed and disintegrated. Fears I had created as a little girl and then as an adult came forward boldly and clearly. They were no longer shaping me unconsciously. I was very conscious of them. I didn't hate them. I actually did my best to thank them.

I also did my best to let them know it was time to leave before I kicked them in the butt, out the door myself.

24

There is a comic sketch where a man is praying to God, saying, "Please, God, please help me win the lottery." God looks down on the man and says, "Please, John, please buy a ticket." I was now John and I was buying that ticket.

It really is not up to us to say *how* things are going to flow our way. It is too easy to put all our attention on that when life is much more creative and capable than we can ever imagine. Being open to the surprise of life can be so much fun when we are in a strong enough place of faith for receiving such. We are all human, though, and faith does waver sometimes before returning as the loyal friend it is.

Already I had been blessed with miracles out of the blue in my life. When I was about to record my first album, a woman I hardly knew came into my life offering me money to support my album. Years later as I put plans into place to begin teaching songwriting in a women's jail, a woman I knew only a little (and someone with a reputation for stinginess with her money) gave me the funds to buy a secondhand van so I could carry equipment to the classes. Of course, the timing of my baby and the publishing contract was also a pretty cool miracle to be blessed with. There had been other perfect and synchronistic events, too.

I knew a bit about miracles and not standing in the way of them by putting all my energy on the *how*. The focus needed to be on the *what*, or in this case, the feeling of living in the home. But I still wanted to help life along by increasing the possible options to bring me and this home together. So each week I bought a little ticket in the lotto. There was no need to spend much money, so I just purchased the minimum ticket. After all, you need only one winning game.

Even still, sometimes I felt that my father winning the lotto was a sort of curse, bringing the possibility of winning the lotto into my own reality. Over the years, it was too easy to get caught up in that dream if I was short on money or needed a solution. This closed me off to other possibilities, including just earning the money.

With an awareness of this reliance, I had sometimes challenged myself in the past to not buy a lotto ticket when things were particularly tough, just so I could remain more open to other solutions. I didn't want to dictate how life should deliver my dreams. I wanted to be strong enough in faith to remain an open vessel. Things then flowed to me through other channels, like new opportunities for earning the money or random gifts. However, I knew that for the amount of money I needed to buy the house, buying a lottery ticket was not entirely a bad idea.

There was also fear about actually winning the lotto and the attention it might bring. Ever since I was a teenager and Dad spoke of winning it a second time, I had a running commentary in my mind, shaping the lies or excuses I would say to detract the attention, to hide the fact of a win from others. It wasn't until I was courageously working through my upper limits regarding the dream home that I truly realized this.

One day when speaking with a friend about the house, I found myself holding back an admission that winning the lottery was a possible way that the money would come. I didn't wish to plant the seed in her mind in case I did win it and she guessed. Instead I had a story in my mind, an excuse for where the money came from.

Later that day I questioned myself as to whether I could actually carry such a lie forward, to say it to people I loved. And I knew I couldn't. Speaking the truth was such an integral part of my values that it was time I faced it. For the first time since I was a young teenager, I considered what it would be like to actually tell the truth if I won some money. It was a revelation to even consider it, having been shaped unconsciously by fear for more than three decades. It was liberating.

I asked the fear what the worst thing that could happen was. "Okay," it said. "Some people may be jealous. Some people may gossip." I considered whether those people's opinions shaped me anymore or was I just conditioned over decades to think they did. I realized they didn't. My happiness had not been dependent on the opinions of others for a long time, but the winning-lotto commentary had been on auto-repeat for decades and I'd never turned it off.

If that was the worst thing that could happen, a bit of jealousy and gossip, what was the *best* thing that could happen? Elena and I would be living in our beautiful home! It was time to focus on that question instead. What was the *best* thing that could happen?

Suddenly a veil lifted and the thought of winning the lotto could start to be seen as a positive thing, a wholly positive thing, without the taint of fear and reprisal. There was so much more I wanted to do besides buy the house. Go to New York, help a friend with her house deposit, buy Mum a new car, send a friend and her family on a holiday, support the dreams of a few people I knew who were already showing incredible courage but needed some help. Of course, I didn't want to win *too* much. I hadn't broken through that upper-limit barrier *completely*, but at least I could finally see winning some money as a marvelous thing.

That night I had a dream I had told the lie, saying that some amazing business deal had come my way, enabling me to buy the house. *It's out there now*, I thought to myself in the dream. The lie was out there. I had said it once. There was no going back. Then a sprout-like infection grew from my gums. As the sprouts then grew outward from my teeth as well, I could no longer speak. Even in my dream, I knew lying was toxic to me. Only the truth would bring me peace. When I woke in the morning, I experienced a wonderful feeling of freedom through the courage of speaking the truth.

While still remaining open to the funds coming from any channel, I decided to help the manifestation of winning along if that was how the money was to come. My relationship with my bank was very personal—a little too personal for me to be comfortable depositing my lotto winnings there if they knew that was where it came from. So I opened an account at a bank I didn't like, one I had worked for long ago and would not feel guilty withdrawing the funds from immediately. I could then transfer the money anywhere, without the drawer of the funds being the lottery company. A girl's got to cover her tracks!

Various research was done into ethical investment funds. I downloaded the winner's claim form from the lottery company's site and filled it in as completely as possible. I addressed the envelope and put the stamp on it. All that was waiting now was the ticket number. Really, if you are planning on winning the lotto, you need to be ready for it.

With all that in place, I could now surrender again, knowing I had done my best to open the channel. Whatever way the money was going to come to me would be fine. That house and I belonged together. There would be a way.

As my self-worth grew, my dreams didn't feel unrealistic or unattainable. The big dreams began to feel more exciting than scary. While all of this was happening, my health was also improving. As I grew stronger, I felt much more capable of managing the home. I felt more capable of managing an amazing life.

Okay, God, I thought. *If you want to give it all to me, I reckon I might be alright with that now!*

Sitting, looking out the window at the rainforest on a glorious rainy day, I felt peaceful and quietly excited. So many fears had been conquered. I had been blessed with the perfect lessons to facilitate that release.

The time was coming for big change. Surely.

25

The seasons rolled by. Despite my best intentions and strong faith, I saw winter come and go. Then spring flittered by. All the while I continued to pay rent, in addition to storage costs.

The cottage was furnished and warmly presented. The landlord had put a lot of love into the place. That was obvious and appreciated. But as romantic as living in a cottage in the rainforest sounds, it really was just a very well-decorated tin shed without insulation.

Throughout winter, my almost crippled hands had loaded the fireplace full of wood. It was cozy while the flames danced but freezing the moment they diminished into ashes. Concrete floors were hard work on my feet. The majority of spring was much more tolerable, at least until summer decided to arrive early with a vengeance. It was a sauna.

Anger began building up in me and flowing out. How could I still be in this place, paying rent, when I couldn't even feel comfortable? There were moments of real anger at myself for having been so foolish to let all this time go by while paying someone else's mortgage instead of my own. And all because of some whimsical dream about owning a particularly beautiful house on a hill.

It felt good to be angry, to allow myself the release. For so long I had stayed unbelievably strong in faith, yet nothing had changed in my home situation. The fact that I was growing into a much more confident and self-caring person, old patterns crumbling away, was totally ignored at this time. It didn't matter that I'd been experiencing unbelievable pockets of bliss and gratitude regularly until then either. No. The anger felt great. I had the shits with life, well and truly.

Being realistic, I had needed to live near others. The landlord's home was within sight of the cottage. They often helped with challenges I had. Now that I was feeling stronger physically, I was outgrowing that need. My frustration just needed releasing. Most of it was not really about the house at all. I was always growing within, but the physical stagnation from such restrictions and disabilities was revolting at times.

The heat in the shed became unbearable, making any kind of activity impossible. When it was at its worst, sweat would roll off me and Elena even if we were just standing still. You couldn't do anything productive. If it was a particularly hot day and we were out and about, instead of being able to head home to escape the heat, I would experience dread and try to avoid going there at all. Living in pain and having a young child did not allow for endless active days out, and we couldn't actually avoid heading home most days.

Resentment began building up whenever the rent was due. Instead of being able to find gratitude for how the place had come our way, for the very suitable role it had played in our lives, for the beauty of its surroundings, and for the abundance in my life to even afford the rent, I just felt angry.

I began questioning faith. It felt great to be defiant, like a rebellious child who had enough. What if faith was really just a load of nonsense? What if I had just wasted almost a year of valuable time and money, dreaming about some house that could never be mine? What if the power of the mind was really a crock of shit, and the only way to get things in life was to work your butt off ridiculously hard and earn it? It was freeing to be so angry and to no longer care. I was cranky at life. I was cranky at myself, and I could not have cared less. Emotional exhaustion gave me further permission to wallow in this swirling well for longer than I usually might.

A period of calm followed that release. My habit of being present and finding gratitude lifted me somewhat, though I might have just been calm because I was so empty and drained. Faith had carried me so well, but I was utterly exhausted from being emotionally strong. Remaining completely dedicated to my hope of obtaining that dream home for a whole year had taken all my strength. Enough was enough.

It was time to let go, to stop trying to control the outcome. What more could I do to make the dream happen? Nothing. I had done my best. The price of the house was still out of my league, even with improved income streams.

It was time to buy something I could at least afford before my savings diminished even further, potentially leaving me unable to enter the real estate market at all. I wanted to respect the gift of money earned that was still in my possession and use it more wisely.

Since my income had continued to improve, the bank approved a decent enough mortgage, one that might have enabled me to buy a house. There were other important dreams, however. If I was genuinely going to surrender the house-on-the-hill dream, I could not surrender everything. For so many years previously I had sacrificed much and worked my butt off, both physically and emotionally, to bring my work to a level of success.

What would be the point if I didn't actually enjoy the success? If all I focused on was more work, more success, or paying off the mortgage? I needed a holiday. We were going to New York, with or without my full health. It was now a non-negotiable. I could wait until the Northern Hemisphere's autumn. What I could not wait for was "someday"—undefined and likely to never happen.

Having worked in the banking industry for more than a decade, I had seen the suffocation people experienced if their mortgage was too high. On paper you can prove you can afford things, but life changes. There are unexpected costs. If I was to have a mortgage, I wanted the repayments to be affordable, unnoticeable. I also wanted a pool, to continue building my strength.

What this all meant was that even though I could potentially afford a house, I was not willing to hang myself with a mortgage so high. So it would have to be a townhouse, villa, or an apartment in a facility with a communal pool. I had never thought that living in such close proximity to others with adjoining walls would ever be a consideration. Even so, I was very grateful I could at least afford something, especially with a pool. That expression of abundance did not escape me. It was just the close confines of neighbors when I was a country girl who thrived best with space to breathe that concerned me.

The difference between clarity and disillusion is often only our perspective of the situation. It was time to look at things differently. I still wanted a life. So I had a bit of a yarn with God. It went something like this: "Okay, God, I am going to hand this over. I want to live in the dream house. You know that. I don't actually want to live in an apartment. You know that, too. I want Elena to have a big yard to play in and I need my privacy. *But* if it's for my highest good, I am willing to buy an apartment and live there. I trust that you will lead me to wherever I most need to be since you actually know my needs better than I do myself. I am in your hands. I trust that all will be well and that there are blessings waiting for me, even if I cannot yet find them in the direction I am facing. I am in your hands." I smiled gently, handing the next chapter of my life over to the creative love of God.

With that surrender and a returning sense of harmony, I ventured into the real estate market to find our new home, whatever it was going to be.

26

Peace surfaced by remembering that life definitely knew my needs better than I did. It had heard constant conversations— all the longings and the fears—within my mind and heart, ever since I was born.

As I had reached a place in my life where I genuinely didn't know what to do, I'd had to discover a new layer of courage, allowing a deeper experience of surrender. It was not a clear-cut process to be done once and then mastered. Instead, surrender was a constant unraveling of faith.

With the new depth discovered, I delicately began stepping forward once more. I was willing to trust again, to be led instead of trying to dictate how things were going to flow. Opportunities to surrender control had always been on offer. They were usually disguised as the times I had the most resistance to letting go, when fear was controlling more than faith.

I had been given the choice to keep putting my energy into forcing things to happen, things that were obviously not flowing as naturally as life can. I could have been sucked into the downward spiral even further, refusing to let go because so much time and energy had already been invested, determining that I would find a way no matter what.

I chose courage to try to let go on another level, by saying good-bye to the house I thought *should* be our home. The fun had gone out of any creative manifesting through my unwavering focus and lack of flexibility. It didn't have to be that hard. By daring to surrender and growing even deeper in faith, I found relief. I had woken up in time. My heart wanted me to be happy. That was the bottom line.

There were a few properties with a pool. I looked at them all. They ticked some boxes, not all, but at least some. I was determined to find *something*. Twice I put in offers on small places. Twice I was outbid.

I then found one where I felt I would be able to write from, which was important since I work from home. I put in an offer. It went back and forth briefly and an affordable amount was agreed upon. It was a small home attached to another on the edge of suburbia with a pool. The view was of a lush valley of farmland.

The access to the home was a bit tricky with some stairs and a somewhat steep pathway. My walking had improved. But in the rain, carrying grocery bags with sore hands and not completely confident walking, it might have been a nightmare. I tried to tell myself I could manage. The view was worth it. Having looked at other similar properties, I knew this one would suit me the best.

My mind flashed a former image before me. It was of driving my car through the remote-controlled door into the dream home's garage, where internal access to the home waited. As the dream property had a couple of large gum trees, I could spot it on the hillside every time I drove near the area. The gum trees were a bit of a landmark. Whenever I had gone by at a distance on a rainy day, I had smiled, imagining myself arriving there and driving straight into the garage before heading into the home without any exposure at all to the weather. Now my mind was back there again. It was not a thought I wanted to be having.

I had one day left to advise the agent of my decision. If I said no, it appeared I would have to continue living where I was. There wasn't much else out there. A renewed test of faith was under way. Was I willing to let the little place go, not knowing what lay beyond, risking even more time in the current cottage? Where did these thoughts of the dream home come from? Why did they have to surface now?

I thought I had already surrendered and found semi-peace in the thought of buying the little place. Yet here was life asking me to step out on a limb, again not knowing what was waiting, doing exactly what I had been doing for a whole year, all because my heart remained with the other house. I had done enough and just wanted to move and get settled somewhere.

As I looked outside from the hot cottage at the rainforest (and actually at the new neighbor afar, tending to his supposedly hidden marijuana plant), I knew what I had to do. No, it wasn't to go and get stoned. With a sigh and slight smile, I climbed back onto the faith bus instead. What choice did I really have? At the last minute, my heart had called out to wait, to not buy the other place. My logical and tired mind wanted to, but my heart spoke in the language I needed to hear—through imagery and feelings associated with the real dream. The clarity was undeniable. That little house was not the right home.

The following morning I was reminded of previous guidance I had received. It was from when I was coming through depression and needing to be strong in hope. My heart had whispered to me, "Smile and know." Now those words came before me again. Stop frowning, fearing, or wondering. Just smile and know.

It was impossible to feel fear when smiling. So I did just that and not only felt happier but felt the dream was possible again.

My thoughts were allowed to return to what I genuinely wanted. It was time to stop wasting my energy on looking elsewhere. I had been willing to surrender the dream, only to learn that in doing so, it seemed I didn't have to surrender it at all.

Somehow, some way, I would be looked after. It would be okay. I was still in God's hands, but I was once again a willing passenger on the ride.

27

When growing through times of turbulence, there is definitely power to be harnessed. The renewed, refreshed energy that lifted me was a welcome change from the storms I had recently experienced. The haze was clearing while I felt the previous tension of fear and control leave my body.

Through the daily whispers of nature outside our window, I was reassured of something far greater at work. It wanted my life to be joyous and through the beauty and cycles nature revealed every day, I didn't need to doubt at all. There was a perfect rhythm and flow unfolding.

Things felt clearer. It was all just energy in the end. The house was energy. The dream of it was energy. My emotions were energy. It all came from the same source. I was a part of that source. It was who I was beneath the layers of my humanness, beyond the tangles of the human mind.

To connect with that divinity, that source of all that is, was where the hard work lay. Not because it actually *was* hard work. I was already connected to the source, in my essence. It became hard work because I forgot and disconnected from it through my interpretations of the human experience.

Instead of remembering that what I wanted actually wanted me too, as it was already a part of my energy field, I had wasted my focus and time on trying to force things and, thus, blocked the flow. It was not intentional. It never is. Why would anyone intentionally block the flow of his or her dream? One word sums it up. *Fear.*

It can be called other things, like control, focusing on how instead of what, or lack of self-worth. Really, though, it was just fear in different dialects. I was afraid of my own potential, seeing my dreams become reality, and being as amazing as I actually could be, in all my full glory.

The dream was waiting, formed through years of thoughts and emotions. The work was in getting rid of the blockages—the things that I thought protected me. It meant removing my security blankets, the patterns I had held on to for so long. They may have once helped me, but now had been outgrown. I was being called to release them in order to move forward into my best self.

Feeling guilty for being too happy was one of my previous security blankets. It was formed from some interpretations made in my child mind decades ago to not outshine anyone in the family. If life became too good, I subconsciously drew something to me to shatter the full glory of that goodness, something to take the edge off so it wasn't *all* absolutely perfect. Over time I came to realize it makes no difference who your family is or what they do or say.

We can all feel blessed by learning through one another, but our paths are individual. So if I dared to find the courage and shine, it was irrelevant whether others also chose to do so in their own lives.

My child mind was once terrified of being noticed. The resulting security blanket had been to blend in as much as possible and not attract any unnecessary attention that would risk wrath and ridicule. It was through acknowledging and releasing the need for the security blankets that true healing was revealed.

The more I dared to be myself, including honoring a career path that insisted I be noticed in some ways, the more I healed. In doing so, the easier life became and the gentler I learned to be with myself.

What I needed to remember was that healing brought happiness. It didn't just remove pain and blockages. It lifted me into a higher place of stronger connection with my true self. This carried more than just happiness. It would bring increasing joy when I was ready to allow it. By focusing on that potential, I opened the flow much faster than by focusing on the pain of letting go.

The act of surrender could feel terrifying. It could also be misinterpreted as idleness. However, it was not doing *nothing*, even if it may have appeared as such. I was mastering an act of bravery. When it was time to act, I would be guided more clearly through intuition, a door opening, or a signpost from life.

Some acts of surrender along the way were not necessarily as obvious. A new awareness to an old habit may have been a catalyst. Any willingness to observe myself, lovingly, and to try to assist positive change was an act of surrender. After all, I was surrendering parts of my old, suffering self.

The more I released such aspects of my past, the more my natural radiance could then be revealed. In breaking through upper limits, there were actually two sides to embrace. As well as working through the blockages that currently held me back, I needed encouragement to keep going. The other side, the balance needed, was to not stop feeling the dream entirely, even if the picture of it had been surrendered. That was where my heart rested. I could continue to feel my way into the dream.

It no longer had to be that very house, though of course a part of me still hoped it was. It just had to be that feeling of home. It no longer had to be perfect health, though a part of me still hoped it was. It just had to be that feeling of freedom and ability. The surrender in these cases was giving up the final image and trusting the emotion I wished to experience was still available. It would also reveal itself in the most perfect way suitable to my soul's journey, in the way that would actually bring me the most peace and joy.

Even with the discipline of decades of meditation, I was still human. My mind still insisted on bringing up old stuff on occasions. Sometimes it was familiar. Sometimes a deeper layer was revealed. Either way, the power I gave to those thoughts was still my choice.

By focusing on the blessings and by smiling when I thought of my dreams, my life was indeed blessed moment to moment by more presence. The turmoil and the yearning subsided again.

When I was first diagnosed with RA, I met a man with no arms. He too had once been fit and strong like me, probably much more actually, since he was managing his own farm at the time. His sweater had become caught in machinery, taking his arms with it. Bless him. There are people all over the world who have had to completely surrender their old identities and rediscover who they are now to be.

My own transformation was individual, as is each person's. All change offered a path to learning and potential peace, providing I could stand grounded in gratitude as much as possible.

Being thankful had certainly transformed my life. I was already not the person I used to be, having said good-bye to much of my previous identity. I gave thanks for that courage but also for how perfect all the lessons had been thus far.

I felt grateful for the courage to continue to dream.

28

One of the emotions I had been longing for most was enjoyment in the kitchen again. My health was gradually improving, though the weight gain seemed to continue despite me eating well. Bloating and deterioration of my visual and oral health were also noticeable side effects from the medications I had been taking for some months now.

What they did give me was more mobility, less pain, and, best of all, the ability to imagine health and independence again. Getting in and out of the car seat was a noticeable improvement. I no longer held tightly with both hands to take one step up or down either.

Through the positive increase in my strength, I could at least now reconnect with memories of wellness. I was closer to the possibility than before, but it still felt like a long way away and was not completely believable every single minute. The fact that I had considered moving house spoke volumes in and of itself.

The side effects of the medications continued to become more noticeable alongside the increasing experience of normality returning. The balance was tipping. But in the long-term, there were potentially bigger problems ahead by staying on the medications.

These observations, added to my somewhat returned abilities, renewed my determination to continue improving. As the medications had offered such a welcomed reprieve, I'd been giving myself a little more leeway with the diet. I was still eating very healthy, organic food, but it was no longer focused on beating the disease. It was just about wellness. The obsession with the diet and healing had taken all the enjoyment out of food preparation and consumption. I had been trying too hard.

A renewed sense of determination arose. Readiness for the next chapter arrived. Life continued to guide me dietary-wise. Through trial and error, it had become obvious that some foods were not in agreement with my gut health.

It had been almost a year since I was fully vegan. I had moved past the guilt while still feeling gratitude and compassion to the animals whose lives blessed my health. My heart was still essentially a vegan one, and I hoped to shift the balance back to that direction one day. But for now fish and organic free-range eggs were also a part of my diet. There were no refined sugars or gluten anymore either.

I was feeling drawn to remove or reduce grains. With the right kitchen setup and a creative, inspired mind, it was achievable. There were also enough specialty cafés around for me to be able to eat out at times.

Many fabulous dietary teachers were online, with countless recipes of delicious meals I could prepare, but I needed to be in the right kitchen and have a feeling of fun associated with meals. This would also mean visitors to feed. It is so much more enjoyable to share meals with friends than to prepare divine meals for just one adult and a toddler who could take or leave the special food, depending on her mood at the time. Not that I didn't also do healthy meals just for us. I did. But my vision included sharing the new recipes that I would discover.

The stronger I became, the clearer that vision for a happy kitchen grew. In the cottage, there was no oven, only hot plates and very few shelves. For a year I had been using a couple of boxes for my food pantry, rummaging through them looking for ingredients all the time. Further pain also occurred since almost every action of my hands was still unpleasant. It felt a long way from the comfort and ease my wellbeing needed and aspired toward.

I wanted to see what I was capable of achieving with my health and diet. As my readiness increased, so did the test of patience. Since letting the little house with the view go, I had been peaceful and present more than not. There were still hard days when parenthood exhausted me or a flare-up would happen and I would be rendered disabled. I was doing pretty well, though, on the extended leap of faith.

One evening, my hands flared up the worst ever since going onto the medications. Inside my wrists a raging fire swirled. In the search for release from agony, my fingers almost begged for amputation. Every single pulse gave further strength to the force of excruciating pain. As it built up, I wondered how my body could actually survive this level of intensity.

I was reminded yet again how even pain can bring blessings. It carried me to a place of release, allowing my tears to flow. Unable to do more, I surrendered, resting my hands on a large cushion on my lap. Sobs grasped for escape, flowing at full force once finding release. Weeping through the pain, I acknowledged my exhaustion. I was not well enough to function at full power. All I really could do was be present, trust, and find gratitude in the ongoing healing.

Resorting to painkillers was not common anymore, not for a long while. Time had both wearied and strengthened me. On this particular evening, though, I waited for them to kick in. There was nothing I could do but cry, wait, and let go into the moment. As the tears continued to flow, I finally realized just how much I had needed the release.

A sense of home and a workable kitchen would make an enormous difference on so many levels. I continued to long for comfort and ease. For the first time in my life, I asked my dear father for support. Finally I had reached a place where I could allow him to help, even if he had died some months earlier. "Come on, Dad. I need your help, please. Let's make this happen together," my heart whispered to him. He had loved Elena so unconditionally. I knew he would want the same for her as I did—a home for her to grow up in, one with a large yard to run around in and space inside to play. He loved me too, even if he had struggled most of his life to show it. I loved him and had likewise struggled. Something was shifting. My heart was finally opening further to his love. Not only did I wish for his help for mine and Elena's lives; I wanted to give him the opportunity to help me.

The pain, release, and prayer for help left me feeling quite empty the following morning, in a good way. There was space for new to come through. The flame of hope had air to breathe once more.

29

With every dream I have watched unfold in my life, there have been two common factors that have made them possible: timing and readiness. The combination determined each dream's arrival from the heart into the physical world.

The timing side of it is a trust thing, believing that life is already orchestrating the dream and will deliver it when all the pieces fall into place. This, of course, is dependent on the other factor—our readiness.

Many times I have felt ready for a dream to unfold and grown frustrated, sad, or angry, or all of those, when it hasn't. In hindsight, I became grateful. Better things, better directions, were revealed over time, helping me make sense of why it hadn't happened the way I had once felt it should.

When I was working so hard to become a singer/songwriter, I applied for numerous artists' grants. There was money available for recording, touring, publicity, and whatever else the funding guidelines specified. I didn't actually enjoy performing for the first years. I was playing to the wrong audiences. Added to very low self-worth, it was a challenging road. Despite this, my need to share my message drove me on, even though my energy was in total conflict with the grant applications. Fiercely, I continued trying to control the direction of my career. Needless to say, none of those funding applications were successful.

While doing this, I was caring for dying people. There was already bigger magic at work, even if I couldn't see it yet. No skills in life were wasted. Everything learned along the way was actually a part of my preparation for readiness. This honored the most authentic path for my soul's growth and happiness.

The years with dying people changed my life immensely. The dying taught me how to live, particularly those who were dealing with massive regrets in the process. Eventually, through one of my patients, I met a great woman who helped me secure funding for the songwriting program I came to set up in a women's prison.

Each step of the journey was perfect. Teaching in the jail suited me much more than doing gigs in noisy, unwholesome pubs. In time, the classroom environment led to me blogging and eventually becoming an author and speaker. All of those experiences performing, most of which I dreaded, were actually my apprenticeship into the speaking world. Immediately I felt a great love and affinity with the new role and could incorporate an occasional song into my delivery too. Being able to share my message as an author was also a dream come true and much more suitable to me than slogging it out as a singer/songwriter.

With all those grant applications, when doors remained closed, bigger blessings waited. The experiences along the way were not only preparing my readiness for the dreams I was focused on, but were bringing even bigger blessings and visions to me.

If the house dream had not yet unfolded, it was due to my lack of readiness and it not yet being the right time. Even if I felt I was ready, which I did more and more by the day, I had to trust in the big picture. There was other healing under way, too.

I was enjoying balance with my work now, having learned not to take on more than I could handle or enjoy. I certainly felt in the flow and loved that I was experiencing this in such a way. I was in a place of allowing instead of striving. It was working and felt good. No uneasiness seemed to surface as I continued to grow at a comfortable pace. The balance there felt healthy.

One afternoon soon after, that vision of myself, of balance, changed. I caught my reflection in a shop window and I looked old—not necessarily old in an aging way but certainly old in a tired way. My body wore the posture of three years of pain. My face expressed exhaustion. Where was I? I had thought I was doing very well since the pain had decreased in recent months. Yet looking at my reflection, I saw other pain expressed. I drove home, praying for guidance to reconnect with the lighter part of myself. I was so tired.

It soon became clear to me that I was somewhat burned out by motherhood and the imbalance I had allowed to build there. It wasn't that I didn't love motherhood. I did, enormously. In fact, this role constantly left me in moments of wonder and overwhelming gratitude. Regardless, something had been surrendered unconsciously along the way, something I now realized that I needed.

There was not one moment in my life for adult time that didn't involve motherhood or work. Even time catching up with a couple of dear friends who didn't have children or whose children had grown up was done with my dear little girl beside me. I didn't want to remove such times from my life. They brought joy—but I also needed to allow some space for time-out, for fun conversations, and lightheartedness with just other adults.

Some beautiful friends had already been made in this new chapter. Mostly they were mums of little ones. Whenever we spoke of exhaustion from parenting, there was a mutual understanding and empathy. Offers of help were given. Most of the mums had since had another child and were set in their daily routines. So I hadn't actually taken anyone up on their offer. Instead we cherished the time we all spent together while our children played. We also spoke of our combined visions to help each other out more when the children were a little older.

If I was going to incorporate more adult time into the present, I was going to have to ask for help. This would involve being able to acknowledge and utilize any offers of assistance and justify the need to myself. If it meant paying a babysitter more often, a great woman Elena loved, then I had to do that, too. There was also a gorgeous tribe of women I had met through an online course. I could lean on them if needed. Just acknowledging the need to myself brought relief.

A part of my vision for the next chapter of my life included a great network of local people. As the dream home was in a cul-de-sac, I imagined helping create a sense of community there. Growing fruit trees on the public land in front of the home was one step toward that, hopefully inspiring neighbors to do the same.

Then we could all share in one another's bounties instead of living completely isolated from each other. I also imagined it being a safe place for children to ride their bikes and visit one another's homes easily. It was not difficult to feel enjoyment from that vision.

In the meantime, life was preparing my readiness. It was teaching me how to ask for help. Sure, Elena could go and visit her grandmother and cousins for a weekend every few months, giving me time out even if they all lived a long way away. But I also needed to get into the practice of leaning on local support. I wasn't just going to arrive in that vision of community support one fine day. I had to grow into it.

As the cottage was revoltingly hot, it was not possible to truly offer much support to others yet. The image of being able to do so persisted, and each time it was in the dream house.

My readiness continued to feel closer. Little did I know how much a dream for home could actually represent, how much I would learn about myself and heal in the process. As I acknowledged the imbalance with motherhood, work, and time out, I grew through even more healing. This assisted my return to joy.

There was plenty of laughter with Elena and her friends. And there needed to be space for laughter with adults, and massages, and staring at the ocean without awareness of time, and going out after dark. I needed more adult company. The balance would not only make me a happier person; it would benefit my little Elena, as I would be an even happier mummy.

Life was a perfect teacher. Life wanted me to know genuine happiness and was holding my hand tenderly as it led me there. Only the big picture would reveal just how many perfect experiences and healed layers there were, already helping bring my dreams into manifestation.

I just needed to continue embracing my growth with as much gentleness and trust as possible.

30

By returning to the area where we now lived, an area I had also lived in years earlier, there were many benefits. It was not like when I moved somewhere knowing nothing about the area, other than that I was guided to live in it for a while. It was much easier to return somewhere. The previous knowledge of the area, combined with the life experience gained in the years since, offered much enjoyment. I felt at home in this region, like nowhere ever before.

Another bonus was that I knew some people. Sometimes familiar faces would cross my path and we would stop and chat. It gave me a nice sense of belonging to run into people I knew. There were also old friends I became reacquainted with. Some were busy getting on with their lives and we just reconnected briefly. A few others had never really left my life. With occasional contact over the years, we simply picked up where we left off.

One of those friends was my mate Jeff. We had met 25 years earlier. From the start, we shared a mutual love of adventure and independence. Over the years our friendship had witnessed many changes in each other's lives. Much of this was through letters written, back in the days of pens, envelopes, and stamps. We would always post them to each other's mother's address since we never really knew where the other might be.

When I was working in a pub in England, he had been in Europe. Despite a train strike and no Internet or mobile phones in those days, he still managed to visit me in the little country village. As young children, we had also lived only a few miles from each other before my family relocated. When we met as young adults, it was in a town another 12-hour drive away. It was one of those friendships with many parallels and mutual respect.

As letters gave way to e-mails and our adult lives became busier, our contact became annual phone calls. Every now and then we would manage a real-life catch-up too. Sometimes they were a few years apart, sometimes many more.

The phone calls were our friendship's lifeline. Those couple of hours reconnecting each year brought us both much pleasure, even though we remained on the periphery of each other's lives the rest of the time.

We would talk of our challenges and our dreams, always with ease, honesty, and vulnerability. In recent years Jeff had been dealt some big learning. Similar themes continued to arise from him during our annual conversations. I, too, shared my vulnerabilities. We loved the ease and the complete lack of pressure or expectation that our friendship offered.

Around the time my father passed away, Jeff and I finally caught up in real life again. My mobility had improved enough for me to feel a little more sociable, though I'm sure I would never have declined his suggestion to reconnect anyway. It had been several years since we'd seen each other. Yet there was no fuss, just a big familiar hug and smile, as if we had seen each other only yesterday.

Even with the very talkative little Elena present, we managed a lovely yarn. We spoke of challenges and dreams. There was also talk of our careers, with both of us being proud of the other for achievements since we'd last connected. Knowing each other as well as we did, most of the talk was of things more important to each of us. There was also talk of music, holidays, and relationships.

I shared how grateful I was to be single at that time in my life. Rather than crave a relationship, I was actually giving thanks that I wasn't in one. At the end of each day, when Elena was finally asleep, I could enjoy silence and my own company rather than have to share my energy with someone else. There was nothing left in reserve. Pain and parenthood were exhausting enough. Just a conversation on most of those nights may have felt impossible.

There was also a part of me that simply couldn't be bothered with another relationship. My mojo was long dead, lost in the pain of disease and lack of sleep. Despite my adventures into sexual discovery in earlier years, I found the celibate life actually suited me. I knew many on their meditation paths who had chosen the same. I hadn't chosen mine as consciously as that, but I still felt grateful to be single.

It was a lovely catch-up as easy and flowing as it had always been. In parting, we gave each other a big hug and promised to reconnect sooner from here on since we were now living only about an hour's drive apart.

Elena and I held hands and waved from the veranda as Jeff drove off. He waved back with a smile and disappeared down the driveway through the rainforest. Within a few seconds he was completely out of sight. Within just another couple of seconds, I was hit with a life-changing realization.

It couldn't be. Where had this come from? No, there was no denying it. My heart had burst open. The feelings were real indeed, and they were for Jeff—my old and dear friend. Something had shifted inside me and I longed to be held in his strong arms again, to know this dear man on a soul level.

He was gone, back to his life, and I was left with confusion and terror. How could this be? How could I have been having a conversation less than an hour earlier and felt genuinely honest in my statements about gratitude for single life? What had happened?

His hug was what happened. I felt at home in his embrace. I wanted to let go and lean into it even more, feeling the relaxed mold of our bodies standing there holding each other, for a little while longer, forever.

As quickly as the heart had exploded, old fears rose to the surface. I didn't want a relationship. I didn't want to lose my independence. I didn't want to live with him. On it went. Throughout the afternoon, every argument of resistance rose. Throughout the same afternoon, every argument was soothed with a gentle, reassuring heart, telling me that everything would be okay. I just had to deal with one small step at a time.

As I lay in bed that night, my little girl sound asleep beside me, I felt peaceful and even found myself smiling. This day had indeed delivered some surprises. There were still fears of what may lay ahead, but there was quiet excitement, too. Jeff was probably the only man in the whole world, besides one gay friend, with whom I could allow myself to be completely vulnerable. We already loved each other as mates. We had shared our vulnerable sides, obviously not to the level that a soul love could take us, but we were on our way.

It was with peaceful trust that I let go into a deep slumber. I may not have been ready for a relationship, but I was willing to surrender into the process of growing into such readiness.

The following morning I woke to the news that my father had passed away.

31

While I sat absorbing the news of my father's passing the day after Jeff's visit, little Elena played nearby. When she saw tears in my eyes, she asked what was wrong. I told her that Poppa had died. "Oh, okay," she said and came and gave me a hug before returning to play. Children are so honest and present. We can learn much by observing their reactions.

Sometimes as adults we are conditioned to think we should be grief stricken when someone dies. Of course, this is often the case, though it isn't always. Although I cried as the news of Dad's departure began to sink in, there was no great sense of loss or grief. More tears came, but from the start, gratitude was certainly the dominant emotion.

Elena did have quite a meltdown about a week later after time spent with me in her grandparents' home without Poppa being there. It manifested as a huge tantrum about not wanting to eat lunch. After I stayed with her and reassured her of my love, she eventually exhausted herself, only to quietly state, "I just wish Poppa hadn't died." It was so honest, raw, and real.

As the day prior to Dad's passing had been such a significant one for me, it was impossible to separate the two events entirely. Sitting with those first tears, I also smiled gently. I like to think that on a soul level, Dad knew he could let go knowing that I'd found someone who would care for me, in Jeff. I like to think that, anyway. It makes me smile and remember Dad more fondly.

About a month after my heart-opening realization and Dad's departure, Jeff and I crossed paths again. Elena and I were in his area and had arranged a morning with him. As we sat on his veranda, overlooking a mountainous valley, it was the same as always between us—easy, honest, vulnerable, supportive, and enjoyable. There was no turmoil, not even the slightest distraction from my new feelings. They were calm. It was simply a lovely morning spent with my old mate.

What was different was the nature of conversation. As we normally only connected occasionally and had already done so recently, the conversation went to new topics. For the first time in 25 years we spoke about memories from our childhoods and of our roles within our families growing up. We still chatted with familiar ease. But there were new discoveries about each other that left each of us smiling whilst listening to the other's stories. It felt so natural that at one point I seriously wondered if I actually had feelings for him beyond friendship or whether they had settled down and completely gone.

Since we had last seen each other, there had been some days when I had not even thought of him. So it wasn't an all-encompassing distraction. It was not surprising to wonder if those feelings truly existed at all. I had expected a bit of nervousness or excitement in me, but it was just us, as we always had been.

When the time approached for us to leave, we stood and chatted more near the car. While doing so, he put his arm around my shoulder and kissed me on top of my head. We were so comfortable with each other that the gesture didn't ignite any confusion in me. We chatted some more before he put Elena in her seat and gave her a kiss good-bye. Then we hugged, said our farewell, and I hopped in the car.

Again, I felt normal and comfortable. Yet the moment I started driving off and he was out of sight, the most powerful longing surfaced. *I have to know this man on a soul level.* The intensity of feelings was so incredible that I almost wanted to scream in urgency. My heart was connected in a way that was well beyond my control. It was completely unlike any previous experience of love I had known.

It was also soon after this particular day that I realized my mojo and interest in sex were not quite as dormant as I had once thought. I was not completely dead in that area yet. Some beautiful, fun, mischievous loving would be good not only for my heart; it would also be good for my health. I began catching myself with a cheeky smile when thinking of sharing with him in such a way.

There was a new feeling of gentleness now, a comfortable patience in waiting. I felt peaceful trusting our time would come. It was not there yet. There were things going on in Jeff's life, conclusions he had to come to on his own without my interference. My own readiness was not quite there either. I was growing into it and could only hope Jeff would too. As much as I was aware of how quickly life can pass us by and how painful dying with regrets can be, I also remembered timing is a powerful thing. So while I didn't want to waste time, I didn't want to push things to unfold before their readiness either.

In the meantime, I had to get on with my life knowing he was doing the same. Our individual lessons were unfolding as they were meant. We were both people who made dreams happen. If our feelings were to find synchronicity with each other, then our time would come and it would indeed be a magnificent thing.

Love calls its own shots. In being honest with myself, I knew that I really didn't have any control over how things would unfold, including the timing. Still, I am human and I am a woman. Not only could I allow myself the enjoyment of daydreaming about this gorgeous man; I could also assist my own readiness by being as clear as possible on what felt right.

Time was already healing me. Any fears that surfaced were not like before. This was Jeff. Love would feel safe this time around. We had the foundation of 25 years of love, honesty, vulnerability, and mutual respect and admiration. It would be a beautiful thing.

How much happiness could I allow myself? That was the question. As I continued to imagine my dreams unfolding, including that of me and Jeff together, I realized just how much I had healed over the previous few years. The fact that I even dared to dream of such happiness helped me gauge my willingness and readiness to actually embrace it. It didn't feel so far-fetched now.

It was all beginning to feel more real. It was just a matter of readiness and timing.

32

Sometimes I had to seriously wonder how I could not be living in the dream house yet. My emotions already lived there so comfortably. Other dreams continued to bloom and expand, too.

Having acknowledged the neglect of my personal needs through motherhood and the imbalance created, my dream now included having an assistant or two—one for professional help, one for the kitchen. After all, if I was going to dream and truly believe in the possibilities of manifestation, then I needed to dream the whole thing.

I imagined employing someone who had a love of holistic food and its preparation. There were many foods I still could not cut as a result of weakness in my hands, foods I loved that would be beneficial to my health. Juicing was also still out—too hard on my hands. I purchased a juice regularly when out and about, but daily juicing would be a vital component in my renewed campaign to health. I also loved the idea of someone preparing food for me at home now and then.

The dream of feeding friends myself still existed. It was just that I loved the idea of having my own holistic chef on occasion, someone who would cater to my diet with enthusiasm and creative flair. With an assistant, even just one day a week, my load would indeed lighten. This would enable me to attend more to my own wellbeing, hence offering more momentum for improvement.

New York was still on the agenda. There was only six months left before I planned to go. My fitness and pain levels still needed to improve enormously. Instead of being overwhelmed, an internal shift was under way, indicating I could actually achieve these changes. Simply acknowledging the burnout from motherhood and the need to attend more to my own wellbeing had untangled some blocked energy. Renewed determination arose.

Being so set on going to New York, I had invited a great woman along to accompany me and Elena to assist with child care. Mel and Elena shared a wonderful bond. She was a fabulous woman— not only with child care but also as someone whose easy company I could enjoy. Mel and I reached a mutually beneficial agreement and were both getting excited about the trip, though I knew I still had a lot to get through first.

Searching for the right apartment in New York was based on walking distance to an organic food store. Although I imagined us discovering as much of the city as possible, there might also be days when staying home could feel more appealing. So the right neighborhood was essential. The research online and in books was exciting. With the recent shifts happening within, the fear of not being able to walk well was finally starting to decrease.

I knew I was getting better as I was feeling increasingly frustrated. When I was at my absolute most frail, there was no real energy to be frustrated. Now that I was feeling stronger, there were moments of less tolerance toward the present. As memories and feelings of wellness returned little by little, my body would remind me that I was still in a different place. It was lagging behind my mind's expectations. Each time it reminded me I had limitations, a mild mix of anger and grief would surface—anger at the physical restrictions and grief for abilities absent. I was losing my acceptance of what was.

No longer would I accept this was as good as it was going to get. When one of my readers e-mailed, hoping to hire me for a walking tour in Australia, it hit home just how much I had loved and missed long-distance walking. Naturally I had to decline her invitation. On a recent morning out with Elena, I had been feeling particularly well. After only about half an hour of very slow walking, I was rendered out of action for the rest of the day owing to the pain in my feet. Obviously my ambitions remained somewhat ahead of my capabilities.

Even so, old memories of walking without pain were subtly surfacing, quietly in the background. I started to truly believe I would get through this, particularly with the renewed vigor and dedication to my wellbeing. Of course, all of it could be summed up as my emotional readiness to be well and radiant again.

With only a couple of days until Elena's third birthday and Mum arriving to celebrate with us, I decided to make the most of the child care from Grandma. It was time to get the ball rolling more toward my well-being.

Feldenkrais was something that had been calling me for a while, so I phoned and made an appointment for the following week. The modality worked with posture and movement. As I no longer felt like the old me, I wanted to discover the new me, including how to hold my body differently. I wanted to stand and move like the person I was becoming inside, not as the person I had been, riddled in pain.

There was another area of frustration that was becoming prominent—that of not being able to play guitar. A couple of months earlier I'd had a dream I was playing and singing around a campfire. It was a Johnny Cash song. I can't count how many times that scenario had actually unfolded in my past. Instead of waking disappointed, I felt happy. I had just been given the memory of how it felt to play—and it felt incredible. I had forgotten how much I loved music flowing through me.

Fear stopped me from getting my guitar out straightaway, and when I did, I was still a little nervous. It was actually Elena who had insisted I do it. One day, she was playing her ukulele and wanted me to play despite having never seen me play before. (She did tell me she remembers me playing while she was in my belly and that she used to love it.)

It soon became obvious I was not going to be the guitar player I used to be. Holding down strings was too painful on my wrists. Most fingers on my left hand hardly bent at all anymore to offer any variety in chord formations. My right hand, which had developed into a nimble participator of fingerpicking, was now rigid with little control in most fingers. I made some noise for Elena that day but happily put the guitar away again.

The smell of my guitar and the feel of it persisted, so I decided to try slide guitar, changing the tuning of the guitar and resting it flat on my lap instead of under my arm. To a degree, I enjoyed the introduction to slide. I had always loved the sound of it being played well (and usually developed a momentary crush on the slide player for the entirety of that one song they were playing). But my left hand did not have the movement necessary. Even with a slide on one finger, you need some movement in the other fingers to add color. As a songwriter, it was frustrating to get a bit of a tune happening and then have nowhere else to take it. Again I put the guitar away.

Little determined Elena wouldn't have it and persisted in me getting it out now and then. We would make up songs with her accompanying me on the ukulele, tambourine, clapping sticks, drum, harmonica—or all of them at once. On one particular occasion, I started singing a new song, an adult song, not a toddler one as I'd been doing. That feeling of creating through trust by just singing whatever came out of my mouth excited me again.

My voice was different—stronger, clearer. It felt amazing to honor its expression. I *had* to be able to play again. I just had to. There were new songs waiting. People had suggested I learn other instruments, but it was the guitar I loved most, the connection with the instrument resting near my heart.

Although parts of myself and my identity had changed dramatically over the years, it seemed that walking and songwriting with guitar were not done with me yet. If I could imagine and feel myself doing those activities, then surely I could pull myself forward and find the solution to breaking through the disabilities currently present. There had to be a way.

Silently, I sent myself some loving encouragement. *You've done well, and the best is yet to come.*

A new vision of myself was forming and I loved what I was seeing.

33

It seems there is no stopping momentum. The closer we grow to readiness, the more signposts indicate that change is coming. This was certainly the case now. From that weary extended period of exhaustion, acknowledging the neglect of many of my needs outside motherhood and work, everything began to change. All it had taken was the acknowledgment to myself that I didn't, in fact, have it all under control. This opened me up to change, loosening the solidity around my vision of the future and myself. It allowed the flow for increasing momentum.

I had already grasped the need to feel my way toward wellness by pointing my mind and emotions in that direction. Now life was assisting me with more support. A friend turned up with an article she had read, some new writings about the pathways of the brain and its association to pain. It reinforced the need to continue thinking myself well, even if this reminder was now coming from a scientific perspective rather than a spiritual/emotional one.

The blend of the two was well timed. It supported both sides of my thinking. They were in unison. The Feldenkrais appointment also proved timely. After only 90 minutes with the practitioner, I was walking with much more confidence and flow. With the amount of tension I felt released from my body, it was as if I'd had a 10-hour massage. She also spoke of the theory mentioned in the article my friend had given me in a more personal way with regard to my individual situation.

At the same time, an online course surfaced from a parenting instructor I had admired for some time. Her teachings were aligned with my own parenting beliefs. I had not managed to get to one of her workshops yet, mostly because of babysitting challenges. This new program was not only online, something I could do in my own time; it was also about loving being a mother and honoring my own needs. It was focused on richer relationships with our children *and* ourselves, allowing more fun to unfold in the process. There were many wise reminders about the celebration of womanhood, not just motherhood. It was perfect.

While Mum visited, we enjoyed a wonderful birthday party for Elena in a beachside park. A dozen of her little friends and their parents joined us. A few other friends came too, friends without children or with grown ones. I looked around the group, all happily mixing with one another, and felt blessed. A couple of them had been my friends for a decade or more. Most, though, were new friendships made in the last 12 months since we had moved north. The party was a team effort from most of those there. I had accepted all offers of help. It didn't feel as hard to accept anymore.

That afternoon, Mum banished me from the very hot cottage so I could join two of my friends for lunch, child-free. As we sat in a lakeside restaurant enjoying healthy food, the three of us shared funny stories about past behaviors and actions—stories that belonged with our younger, insecure selves with whom we could now laugh compassionately. As each story unfolded, life felt lighter. By the time I returned home, I had connected with a feeling of normality and ease that had been absent for too long.

The following evening, I headed off to a movie on my own—after dark and all. Knowing that Elena was being loved and cared for by her doting grandmother allowed me complete freedom to relax. It was a good movie, one that triggered all the right emotions. Thank goodness. When you only get to the cinemas for one movie per dark age, you want it to be a good one.

Driving home, I finally realized I had wanted to get healthy again for Elena and for all the people who loved me. I had thought I was trying to get better for myself, but I actually wasn't. I had wanted to be a better mother. I had wanted to inspire people through my own learning, helping their recovery. I had wanted to be out of pain, but I hadn't really been pulled forward by the things that I most needed.

Now I was willing to do that. My desire for walking, music, and fun rose to prominence. All the other reasons still existed, but now I wanted to get better for reasons that would actually gift my own life. It was time to get better, for me. I finally loved myself enough to do that.

When living by trust and intuitive guidance, life's signposts become impossible to ignore. So it was not surprising the home situation continued to deteriorate around this time. As the cottage was so unbearable with the heat and I had been a good tenant for more than a year by now, I requested a reduction in rent. It was granted, but not before a condescending reply about how good I had it there with no contract. It had actually been a mutual blessing for both sides and had served us all well. Obviously it was just time to go.

If it wasn't the heat and rent cost, it would have been something else. My energy was no longer aligned with living there. Discontent had been building for too long. The yearning for home existed for decades but had gained enormous strength in the previous 12 months, to a point that it was never going to accept being silenced again.

I did my best to find peace in the time remaining there. Confidence for change grew. The time to go approached. Just where was I going, though? That was still the question.

34

Life was questioning just how willing I was to raise my expectations for myself, to acknowledge my own worth. With all of those years I spent meandering, I never imagined that my longing for my home would ever rise to such prominence. Better still, I never imagined the search for it would teach me so many beneficial things.

Most days I was still pretty strong in faith, smiling as I continued to imagine us living in the house on the hill. Deep down in my heart, the light of hope for it never fully extinguished. Other days I was not so strong, and each time the heat pelted down into the tin shed, my ability to endure further waiting was tested.

It was not that the previous efforts of surrender were not real or total. They were in their moments. My heart surrendered entirely each time, returning to a place of trust in the unfolding pace. But in being called to be my complete best self, something my heart had actually asked for, my faith had to continue deepening until it was absolute.

The ebb and flow of my energy and focus revealed a layer-by-layer unfolding. Each occasion brought a deeper experience of surrendering to the divine and a molding of more solid foundations of trust in the big picture. But it *was* one layer at a time, and in between, my frailty and humanness were tested.

For so long I had been such a dedicated servant to faith, truly believing I could own that magnificent home on the hill. Yet every day I continued to live in a hot shed with people telling me what rules I had to live by.

I tried to use my feelings for Jeff as an example for my dream of home. In this case, there was no doubting the act of surrender. He would be my partner one day or he would be the catalyst for me in finding the right man. No turmoil had arisen at all in that regard. Thoughts of him still accompanied me. But instead of causing impatience or frustration, they inspired me. Every new thought of him gently prized my heart open a little more. There was no urgency, only gratitude for the process unfolding. I wished I could manage my longing for home in the same way.

From moment to moment I did my best to pull back into the present. This was more often than not, but there were other times when I just could not stand it anymore. It was those moments that found me online perusing more real-estate sites and reasoning with myself about the potential benefits of each one. I didn't want to put all my efforts into looking at places my heart did not want, particularly when I had found the home my heart did want. But I was *so* tired. My desires for the kitchen and our own space were becoming unbearable. It was driving me crazy.

It was rare to find a detached house with a pool in the region and price range I was seeking. So when one presented itself, we went to see it in a flash. I then saw why it was the lower price. There was a lot of work to be done. I put in an offer, telling myself we could do it up over time. The pool was nice. The backyard was private. A phone call from the agent later that day informed me of other interest in the property. I would have to raise my offer. I did.

A little while later, something clicked in me. Things were not ideal where we were living and I certainly had to get out soon. I thought about the latest house and how much effort it needed to turn into a home I could love. It was tiresome to imagine. It was excitement that I wanted to experience with the move, not dread or resignation.

Life was also offering me a lesson in self-worth. I could possibly buy that place and do it up in a couple of years, but did I really want this house? I wanted a home, yes, but at what price to my happiness?

It reminded me of all the years I spent in banking jobs. My heart was not in that career at all, yet I moved from town to town and bank to bank for about 15 years. Even though I dreamed of something better, I continued to settle for what I knew, not what I wanted. It was only when the pain of betraying my heart became too much that I was finally brave enough to leave that industry forever, venturing onto the artist's path and to where my heart truly lay. It was also where life rewarded me for that courage.

A similar lesson unfolded now. I had already lived in old homes in need of work, mostly rentals. Settling for houses that were not always particularly nice or well kept was something I had often done. Even though it didn't fit who I now was or who I wanted to be, it was familiar. I could go down that road again because at least it would be our own place with no rules from landlords or residential complex managers. The agent asked if I was willing to raise my offer again.

The feeling of living in the house on the hill came back. It felt so *incredibly* lovely. The house was clean and comfortable. At that moment, I realized I had to just keep hanging in there. I didn't like where we were currently living, but I was also done with living in neglected houses. I loved myself enough to recognize I did indeed deserve to live somewhere comfortable.

It was with this new sense of self-worth that I let the other house go, removing myself from the bidding process.

35

On a gorgeous Sunday morning following this raised level of self-worth, Elena and I headed to an artists' market in a park by the beach. Visiting markets was something I had yearned for when she was younger, when I couldn't walk more than a few meters. Accepting the offer of a wheelchair at an airport around that time had brought immense relief from pain. That experience led to my contemplation of buying one, along with hiring a caregiver, just so Elena and I could enjoy some markets together. This was a particularly happy day, being able to now walk through a market.

My realization the previous day that I was done with crappy homes elevated my mood even more significantly. No longer was I going to find romance in the idea of rustic if that meant cold drafts blowing through the gaps in old homes. I didn't have to settle for vermin keeping me awake at night either. Grabbing buckets for a leaking roof was also too familiar and no longer acceptable. Instead of reasoning that I was still living better than millions of people in the world, I recognized I lived in a society that offered greater comforts than I had sought or expected.

So despite the current challenges in finding a home, I was no longer willing to settle for anything less than I deserved. Comfort and ease were crucial. Finally I could *feel* my worth, not just affirm it. I was going to live somewhere perfect for me and Elena, no matter what. Although I felt happy, I felt fierce, too. My resolution to live the way I deserved and wanted increased in strength.

As the sun shone down, we browsed the market slowly, eating frozen ice pops of pure fruit. Then Elena enjoyed the playground while I gave my feet a rest, sipping a chai in the shade of a pandanus tree and watching her play. I felt wonderful and so blessed to be well enough to enjoy markets again. The ocean looked glorious. A busker sang out happy old tunes. It was one of those perfect moments in time—light, easy, happy, just as a Sunday morning should feel.

As my mind drifted away, a simple realization hit me. From the moment I had seen the house on the hill, I had assumed I would buy it furnished. I had been so ill that it seemed the best choice. The idea of going shopping for furniture, since it would have involved more than three steps, was too much.

When I had been designing the interior of the house in my head, it involved influences of the existing furniture I would acquire with the purchase. Now I realized just how much that image was stopping me from truly feeling at home there.

Shifting furniture around was also not likely to be an easy job for someone who still had to use two hands to turn a key. Practical things that were simple for able-bodied people or those with support often left me puzzled and scared.

When I imagined buying the house empty, it felt like home in a way that it had not previously. It no longer felt as scary. Over the 12 months of growing into this dream, so many fears had surfaced, all of which I dealt with one step at a time. Plenty of overthinking had been indulged. It was all just more layers of fear being dissolved.

Was buying the house empty the missing factor? I wondered. As I continued to imagine it with just our belongings, it felt easier. One sofa and three lamps might not quite furnish the large living area, but what fun Elena and I were going to have in creating a home together, shopping for furniture that suited us—simple, happy stuff.

Now all I had to do was allow the money through to buy it. Despite the reduction of pain, I was still too exhausted from it to contemplate new ways to bring the funds through. The energy of renewal had not yet completely replaced survival mode. Seeds I had planted through the previous years of work still increasingly supported us. But other than maintaining that existing flow of my business with small steps forward, there was not much else physically that I could do.

What I *could* continue to do was the real work—the inner work. So I continued to strengthen my faith and the belief I was being led to the perfect home. Faith works miracles much better than logic.

36

Every two or three steps forward that I took through trust led toward the goal of home. Every effort I made into looking at other homes, trying to convince myself that they would be okay, felt like a step backward. It had become a bit of a wobbly walk forward at times, with a little sidestep and backward step thrown in now and then.

As I worked through the pendulum swings of faith and fear, a unique dance was being created. Rather than beat myself up over dancing to my destination, instead of pacing with solid, focused consistency, I tried to smile compassionately at myself. None of us are strong and focused every single day, particularly when trying to attract miracles through faith alone. Being willing to allow my humanness to exist extended my patience.

When I could, I always returned to faith, with every occasion unveiling a deeper experience of it. Sometimes I prayed for help, which was separate from faith. There was no need for prayers of help with faith, as in that space there was *already* trust and certainty.

Prayer has many faces. Those of thanks and devotion are different from those asking for specific outcomes in our day-to-day lives. Both kinds can bring tears. One is of overwhelming love for the divine and our own desire for such connection. The other is created through intense fear and desperation. Both kinds of prayer still request guidance. The main difference is that the prayer of gratitude and devotion is a calling from the soul. It does not come with conditions. The prayer of desperation for changes in day-to-day life originates from fear from the mind.

It was a blend of both prayers that I turned to when truly scared. While I still felt gratitude often, I knew that no dream had ever come about without help. In quiet moments of prayer, the help I most asked for was strength. I also prayed for connection with my own self, my divine self, who knew the power of faith and timing. I prayed for readiness. I prayed for home. Then I let go of it all and, once again, stopped asking for anything other than the strength to be present and trusting.

As my breath deepened in quiet moments of meditation or prayer, there was no craving, only connection. All would be well. It already was. Life reassured me through feelings of peace.

Despite the frustration I had created along the way, joy was never too far from my side. During the worst of the illness, the slightest reprieve of pain caused joy. Those feelings of freedom, even if only for very brief moments in between intense pain, often left me in unexpected states of bliss and gratitude.

As a result, my awareness of the feeling of joy had grown incredibly stronger in the last few years. It wasn't only an imagined ideal. It was a firsthand experience. Although I was still going through fear and frustration in my humanness, I found myself in pockets of joy at other times.

The more presently I lived, the more stillness I created, the more alive I felt and more open I became to life's blessings. Even so, when I *was* present, there were no actual cravings for those blessings. They belonged in the future or were shaped by the past. In presence, there was no craving or aversion. There was peace. Having grown tired of the pendulum swing, I made presence the real destination.

It was in such a state that I realized what a wonderful teacher food was proving to be. It not only represented health but self-kindness and the intuitive expression of my body. I had to pay close attention to my diet while remaining open to my body's evolution and the guidance it gave. No longer was I fixed on a set eating regime for life or having to categorize myself through that.

I knew I was on the right track when I found myself confidently dreaming of doing something "normal" again, something that was not limited with disabilities. A few days later, after such a relaxed state and a little lenience on the diet, increased pain would remind me I was still some way from being out of the woods completely.

Diet was also having a noticeable effect on my longing for a home. It was not only creative cooking and sharing that I yearned. Diet was teaching me self-love on a whole new level. Finding my home shared an unbreakable link with it. The two had joined forces, calling me to rise up, step forward, and treat myself with the immense amount of love that I deserved.

Life was no longer telling me to eat well because I had a disease. It was calling me to eat well simply as an expression of love toward myself—because I loved myself enough to do so. That was both the challenge and the yearning.

I was still struggling to get creative in the kitchen where we were living, though I did okay some days. Mostly, stagnation was increasing. Browsing recipes and diets that supported autoimmune diseases inspired me at the time, but to transfer that excitement back into my own kitchen was a struggle.

I carried on one day at a time, formulating new ideas in my head about possible recipes. My challenge, besides not enough love and time given to more creativity in food preparation, was that my old staple recipes didn't fit anymore. They contained foods I no longer ate. I needed happy time in the kitchen trying out new recipes, finding which ones felt natural and easy for me to throw together regularly. With the intention of creating new dishes, ones that would incorporate an abundance of nutrients, color, and taste, I began small experiments in the current kitchen. I was still terribly uninspired, but a little more determined.

One particular day, as I fumbled through the boxes that substituted pantry shelves, frustration exploded. Every movement of my hands ignited pain. It was not as intense as it had once been, but they remained delicately tender. Lifting glass jars felt like carrying a 44-gallon drum. Even medium-size jars had to be lifted with two hands, while other ingredients in the box collapsed on top, creating further agony. By the time I had found only three or four items to use, my hands were on fire again, extinguishing any remaining enthusiasm.

Having ingredients easily accessible and refrigerator shelves bursting with fresh food and color became essential. *I'd had enough.* Something switched in me, as my intention to prepare a colorful, divine meal was thrown out the window. The frustration and yearning for home, and in particular a workable kitchen, became too much.

That night, Elena and I ate our substitute dinner: chocolate-banana ice cream. It was still relatively nutritious, made with frozen organic bananas, cacao powder, maple syrup, and macadamia butter. But it wasn't what I wanted to be preparing.

The pain of staying where we were *now outweighed* the pain of not living in the house on the hill. The yearning for the dream home had taught me great resilience for more than a year, but it wasn't enough anymore. The pain of staying somewhere without a comfortable kitchen was now greater than my desire for *the* house. I really did have to let it go.

My heart ached and tears flowed. I had done my best, my absolute best. Time and again, I had come up against the challenges of living by faith and daring to constantly surrender to it. There was not one ounce of emotional strength remaining to stay focused on the dream.

It truly was time to move on. Somewhere within me I would find my way back to trusting in the big picture. That evening, though, I was just too sad to find any positive reasoning, faith, or even hope. It was too painful trying to make the dream happen any longer. More so, it was too painful living where we were without a decent kitchen and a sense of home.

Once Elena was asleep I returned in a somewhat resigned state to the real-estate pages. This time, there was no feeling of resistance. Exhaustion squashed any strength for that. I knew I had done my best to attract the house I wanted. With a weary heart, through the pages I scrolled.

Perhaps I could have strived harder physically to make the dream house happen, increasing my income by saying yes to more. That had already been me, years ago, and those efforts had paid off. They had especially taught me about life and imbalance, and how much more important the inner work is.

Regardless, I didn't have it in me to force and strive anymore. Not only was I not that person now; I was the mum of a toddler and still living with physical health challenges every single day.

I had done my best. I needed to give myself a break by acknowledging my possibilities in the current moment.

It was time to get back to the blessings of what I *could* do, not what I couldn't.

37

Things felt a little easier when I awoke the following morning. The pain of trying to force the outcome, of trying to control it all, was shifting. Through the state of presence I had come to know, the guidance I needed had come. It was time to truly let go. All would be well. Somehow, all would be well.

I arranged the inspection of a villa for later that day. I was heartbroken, but accepted it had to be done. I needed a new beginning, a new kitchen, renewed energy to support my health and healing journey. Above all else, I really *had* done my very best in focus and faith.

Elena and I headed out for our haircut appointments. My hairdresser was a wonderful person and, as usual, it was a delight to chat with him. By the time we arrived back at the cottage, my mood had lightened.

There were still a few hours left before we had to head out again to inspect the property. As Elena stood happily playing with her dollhouse and I stared out the window, the phone rang. It was my dear friend Jeff. He was nearby and did I feel like a visit from him?

I couldn't have asked for a more perfect sign of encouragement. It left me feeling reassured by God that everything would be okay. By giving me such a nice surprise to lighten my day, life told me I was still being looked after. It would all be fine.

It was probably a couple of months since Jeff and I had seen each other, but we had spoken on the phone a couple of weeks earlier. It had been a typically long conversation of philosophy and sharing. Every time we connected, our friendship grew closer. The increasing depth of conversation was impossible to ignore.

With that particular phone call, we had spoken at length about male and female energy. It was an inspiring and intelligent yarn, leaving both of us more connected to our individual roles and sexuality. It also left us even more understood by each other. I found myself sharing thoughts with Jeff about things I had pondered over the years but had never fallen into the right conversation to vocalize.

When we came onto the subject of our mutual and previously unknown to each other love of ancient history, our talk shifted gears even further. It ignited an ability to express my femininity in ways I'd never done before. On the surface, it may have just sounded like two friends having a yarn about strong characters in ancient history and the polarities of masculine and feminine energies. Below that, however, were a bond and an understanding being born that brought me a sense of true homecoming and comfort. It felt incredibly easy and safe to share my truth and vulnerabilities.

The visit was just as pleasurable—even more so as I could enjoy his physical presence too. As we delved deeper into relationships and our ideals, we remained in the safe position of being just friends.

It would have been premature to force things beyond that. It was comfortable and right as it was. I felt no need to declare my feelings since the strengthening of our connection was already unfolding. There was no denying the enjoyment we were both experiencing through our conversations. That felt like enough for now.

After our farewells to Jeff and a gorgeous big hug from him, Elena and I traveled up to look at the little villa. Jeff's visit had certainly brought pleasure in itself. And through that little surprise, one of the best I could have asked for, life had gifted me with reassurance at a time I most needed it.

The villa was fine. It was accessible. The small mortgage would be easily affordable. A line of tall trees, offering privacy and a natural outlook, hid the back fence. Such greenery would help my writing process. Nature always inspired creativity. The side fence joined a lovely park where birds sang at good volume from the trees above. Swimming would be easily accessible in the communal pool and the complex was not too large. The villa also had a great backyard for Elena, one that was safe, protected, and visible from most of the house.

My offer was accepted a couple of days later, after some negotiating back and forth. The pest and building reports were arranged. My mind often returned to the house on the hill, but I chose not to linger there. Now it was time to make it as easy on myself as possible. I was blessed to be able to afford any place at all. It was a nice little place at a good price.

Each day brought me a little more peace. It would take a month or so for all of the legalities to go through, but at least the wheels were turning. We would at last be moving on.

38

In acknowledging the recent imbalances with my own needs, it was time to have some Bronnie time. A dear friend asked me what I would most like to do and what she could do for me.

So with Elena in the wonderful care of Mel, we honored my wish. It wasn't to go wild. It was simple and uncomplicated. A restaurant I knew of further up the coast was the first port of call. On a perfect summer's night, we dined outside on divine, fresh, healthful food and some rather scrumptious raw desserts. Then it was south to another favorite café for a cup of chai.

The thing I most wanted then unfolded. We simply drove to a beach closer to home and sat on the sand, under the stars, listening to the waves, and talked. This friend and I had been mates since we were girls of 11 years old. It was impossible to count how many hours we had spent over the decades sitting at various beaches, philosophizing under the stars with the waves soothing our souls. It felt normal and wonderful to be doing so again.

Then a major achievement unfolded as I stood up from the sand. I actually stood up, on my own, with nothing to pull myself up with. Also, it being my birthday that night, standing was the best present ever to receive. It opened a whole new world for me.

The following morning I was able to sit down with Elena wherever she was playing, not just near the lounge to pull myself up by. The confidence to get myself down and up independently had at last been returned. Elena was puzzled at first, but we both loved it. When we wrestled around, laughing and pretending to tickle, both of our hearts smiled in glee.

It still amazed me after three years that this gorgeous little being called me Mummy. Sometimes when watching her play or listening to her telling me something, my heart would explode in love. Tears of gratitude surfaced without announcement. This was my life now. I was this little girl's mother. All of those years of moving around, all of that lonely restlessness, all of the pain and suffering, was leading to this life—one of unconditional love and the blessing of guiding this divine little girl.

She was not only my daughter; she was a witness to my recovery. As we wrestled around that morning, I experienced complete bliss—true, unlimited, pure happiness. I was coming through it. There was no going back.

I repeatedly chose to focus on what I *could* do, unwilling to be shaped by the identity of a sick person anymore. Both the illness and the dream for home had allowed me to examine my consciousness often, preparing me to know my fullest potential. To truly fulfill my destiny, to fall into synchronicity with the divine plan for my life, I had to step up and own my potential without embarrassment, shame, guilt, or fear.

For all of those years long ago I had roamed around, moving from town to town, and then more tightly through house-sitting, from house to house. That lifestyle gifted me with an immense amount of life experience and I wouldn't trade it for anything. It helped me become who I am. Still, it was hard at times and a very isolating lifestyle. It also kept pain partially subdued or at a distance, as no one could get too close for too long.

Through those years of emotional healing, the need for home had continued to grow. I was much more settled and grounded in myself now. I was a whole different person. Because I also had a little girl to think about, my search for home was very different. If I was still on my own, perhaps I could have been happy with an apartment within walking distance of healthy food, a café strip, a good bookstore, a decent cinema, and a beach or lake. But I wasn't on my own and I didn't want to be.

Even though it was proving much harder to manifest the kind of home that I wanted to provide for Elena's childhood, I found myself actually feeling grateful for the challenge. In wanting her to have space to run around in, I would also be blessed with earth to connect to, birds to serenade me, and nature to be inspired by. These were all things my soul needed, too.

It felt fantastic to have given up the fight for the house on the hill—and that's what it had become. There was newly found space within from knowing another option existed. Secretly, I did continue to hope that a miracle would land *just in time*. Previously, I had experienced miraculous reprieves at the very last minute. God is never too late. If the dream house was meant to be, then it would be. Perhaps I would still buy the villa, as an investment then. I didn't dwell on the idea, but it was there.

The time came to pay a holding deposit on the villa. The funds were transferred to the agent, not with excitement but relief. At least that was a better feeling than dread.

Without any conscious intention, I phoned the travel agent. Like the house situation, I had my ideal scenario imagined. It did not include flying economy class to New York. My publisher had blessed me during that trip to London a couple of years earlier with a more spacious class. It took no time to get used to that. So like the house on the hill, I had high dreams of traveling comfortably. Also like the house dream, I now wanted to focus on gratitude and the current opportunities presenting themselves.

So the day I paid the house deposit, I also bought our economy tickets to New York. It was happening. That dream of "one day" had a confirmed date. I looked forward in peace and with a tad of excitement. We were going to New York! This dream was made true, by taking action and transferring the trip from the "one day" basket to the "I'm making this happen now" basket. Life was too short to dally any longer.

I had seen enough people die with the pain and anguish of regret. One thing was for sure. I was not willing to be one of them.

39

One of the best ways that life can pull you out of your own thoughts is to provide you with an opportunity to serve others. Even though I had cared for several dying people in years gone by, it had been a long time since I felt capable of serving other than as a mother. Life had been teaching me how to receive instead.

A couple of opportunities to serve presented themselves out of the blue. I was mentoring a potential author, but owing to blocks in her, I had to step up and become more of a life coach than a writing mentor. It served us both well, allowing her wisdom to finally start flowing into a book.

A dear friend also asked if we could do some energy exchanges. I would help edit some of her articles and nurture her writing skills. In return she would spend some time with Elena when I needed some solo time, perhaps for a massage or some other act of kindness toward myself. It would be a balance of serving and receiving, one I would definitely enjoy as the needs arose.

I wanted to serve again, to reconnect with that part of myself. Around this time I received the news that Mum had fallen off a stepladder and had a broken wrist. The freedom of my lifestyle and being able to work from anywhere or take a little time off unannounced was truly a blessing. Elena and I packed ourselves up and headed off to look after her.

Before we left, I had a surge of energy enabling me to pack up a lot of the cottage. It made things more believable. We *were* moving on soon. While we were at Mum's, contracts were exchanged on the villa. It was okay. The fight was over. I existed in a place of acceptance. Whatever was going to be would be just fine.

It was lovely to be able to care for Mum. Her wrist had been broken badly, requiring surgery for the insertion of a plate and six screws. Her tailbone was also broken. She resisted painkillers as much as possible, but became overwhelmed by the intensity of it. As a result of the medication, she was sleeping a lot on and off through the days. It was strange to see such a vibrant, dynamic woman so vulnerable and accepting of help.

We cheered Mum on as best we could through her initial healing. My siblings all lived nearby to help her out before and after our stay. It was a special time to be able to look after Mum for a change. She could bathe and use the toilet herself but was unable to dry off properly from the shower without assistance. Cooking meals was also out, so I took on that role. Doing the washing, teaching her stuff on the computer—in any way I could, I helped.

There were many beautiful conversations between us, as well as much delight with Elena and her enthusiastic storytelling. Still, as early evening rolled around each night, I found myself in complete exhaustion and throbbing pain. I was much better than I used to be, but the extra exertion truly brought home an awareness of my remaining limits. With each level of physical improvement, my mind had jumped ahead, leading me to believe I was more able than I had thought. The improvements were wonderful, but the lessons in self-care were still under way. A week was all I could give, and Mum insisted that there was plenty of other help available through family and friends. She also wanted us to get home to our own life.

There was sadness in saying good-bye. Over the years, I had come to dread the sight of her waving in the driveway, putting on a brave face every time I left for another chapter of my life. Yet she was an evolved and wise woman, also knowing that I had to live my own life. It was good to get back up north. Our routines and activities were already structured around my capabilities.

A visit to the rheumatologist confirmed the improvement in my health. My blood tests showed that things had clearly changed significantly. When I asked if we could now reduce the medication, he looked at me as if I were the best comedian in the world. With a big smile and a kind heart, he shook his head no. Hearing his further explanation, I understood where he was coming from. I was just so eager to rid my body of the toxicity of the drugs. I was not so keen, however, to return to the crippling levels of pain I had known for too long. So I accepted his guidance with a quiet determination for such reduction down the track.

There were now four weeks until the property ownership was complete. I knew it was happening and felt very present and trusting with the process of how things would unfold.

While sitting in and commenting on a gorgeous chair at a café a few days later, I was informed they actually had another, very similar one for sale. It was a big, comfy chair, with arms and a very high back, covered all over in a patchwork of colorful velvet squares. It was love at first sight. Gleefully, I paid a holding deposit. They were happy to wait until settlement to deliver it. I allowed myself to imagine the chair in the little villa. I could make anywhere feel like home.

My relationship with Elena was now stronger than ever. Not being so distracted or overwhelmed by pain allowed for more patience and fun. She was clearly an amazing little being, constantly reminding me of how much I could learn through her simple delivery of profound wisdom. It was encouraging to see my efforts to parent consciously paying off. She was indeed a free-spirited soul and I would continue to do my best, allowing the full expression of herself to be. We were having ever-increasing fun together, as well as some remarkable conversations. Of course, she was still a gorgeous, vulnerable little three-year-old girl, too, needing lots of her mummy's kisses and cuddles.

One night when we were at Mum's place, I had watched her sleep as I often did. The difference this time was that she was sleeping with her grandma. The light of the full moon was shining gently into Mum's room. Both of them were in deep sleep—a grandma in her late 70s and her dear little granddaughter beside her. The evening was incredibly peaceful, bathed in soft moonlight, offering me a moment of complete purity. My heart ached with love for them as I stood in the doorway, watching their gentle, restful breathing.

As I lay down to sleep that night, I thought of them in the bedroom on the other side of the house, deeply peaceful in their sleep and in their love for each other. Once my feet were elevated, pain eased, allowing me to let go easily. Before I drifted off into my own enticing slumber, I took note of my life. It was good. It was actually fabulous. Yes, there were challenges—lessons in self-love shaped in one way or another, as there are for us all. But I had come a *long* way from the person I once was.

Whenever I asked the disease what it wanted to teach me, I broke through another layer of self-discovery as further insights were revealed. There was great perfection in the way my healing had been offered to me through RA. Despite exhaustion and pain, I lay there in a place of incredible thanks.

That flowing gratitude accompanied me back up north. Instead of frustration or exhaustion, I returned in a state of peace. When I consciously searched inside of myself, I came across no resistance whatsoever in that moment. It was like I was a supple young tree, grounded enough to hold on, but adaptable enough to lean whichever way the breeze would blow me, without resistance or fear.

With a trusting and happy heart I pondered where the wind would blow me next. Then I was no longer a tree, but a soft green leaf, letting go completely, enjoying the dance without knowing the destination. Wherever I would end up, it would be a gentle landing.

In the meantime, I continued to exist in a state of presence. There was really only one emotion with the present so unaffected, and that feeling was joy.

40

I couldn't live in my conscious dreams and longing all the time. Life continued to unfold and wanted to be lived. There were children's birthday parties, playgroups, visits to old and new friends, fun excursions, work, and general survival duties of grocery shopping and kitchen time.

As the clock ticked down, the house settlement date grew closer. Whenever I chose to consciously contemplate the reality of moving into the villa, there was acceptance. My heart experienced no excitement, but it had given up resistance. I could even find a little sentimentality. The villa was bought with the earnings from years of hard work and sacrifices as an artist.

Through the massive processes of letting go over the past few years, facilitated mostly by RA, I had indeed transformed into a new person. The intense and prolonged physical and emotional pain had ensured this, shaking off numerous old beliefs and habits. So I *could* settle for the villa, but it might not actually fit me forever. Comfort, abundance, ease, and a true sense of home were my magnets.

Love for myself was also now genuine and comfortable. I was no longer ashamed to be happy or embarrassed to experience abundance. The opinions of others that had shaped my past were stale and obsolete, having slipped somewhere into complete irrelevance somewhere along the journey. Freedom was mine. I had found happiness through a path of immense pain. Happiness could obviously be found anywhere. It didn't need life to be absolutely perfect in every way.

Money was not necessarily a conduit for happiness either, but it could create increased ease and facilitate broader options in lifestyle and self-care. It could be a good thing—a beautiful energy wanting to dance with me as much as I wanted to dance with it.

Walls that had once stood in my mind's way crumbled. Stepping over them, I stood tall and strong in my new reality, one that fit the amazing person I had become. Without fear or discomfort, I stepped up to own my new role.

In the meantime, some quality work opportunities were flowing my way. Although the New York trip was initially a holiday, it would have been madness not to make the most of proximity whilst there. Australia is such a long way away. My lifestyle in the last few years had left me feeling further isolated.

Something in me wanted to be a *part* of New York whilst there. So with complete ease, I nudged gently on some career-enhancing doors that swung open easily, welcoming me forward. There would be plenty of time for leisure. We were there for more than a month, and it *was* also time to step up in my career.

My health enjoyed this new confidence as efforts in the kitchen improved. As well as learning more about my stature through Feldenkrais, I had regular appointments with a new chiropractor. When I had been working with one earlier on the RA journey, there had always been an improvement in my mood, but my health had raged into a downward spiral. In the end, I grew weary of further time and expenses for more appointments. Now things were different. I was working with a doctor whose approach and technique were much more congenial to my body and philosophies. My body responded positively to her healing hands.

More important and beneficial to my recovery than any treatment or improved diet were my thoughts. The absence of guitar playing still haunted me. It came up on days when I wasn't so strong. New songs would surface in the background, reminding me of future possibility.

The lack of ability to be on my feet for long certainly wore me down. When a friend spoke passionately about how wonderful her recent trip away had been and how much she had walked, it took all my strength not to dampen her joy with tears. I held those for when the phone call ended. My heart was still breaking at times.

I longed for the freedom of walking enjoyably again, not just to walk when necessary for as little time as possible.

Life blessed me with a signpost to possibility. One particular morning, I woke with *no* pain in my feet at all. It was almost a foreign feeling, yet vaguely familiar from a distant past. There had not been one day for the whole of the past three years where pain was completely absent. So there was no way I was wasting this day, one that offered a sense of immense freedom, so light and *easy*.

Elena and I had been doing some swimming in a couple of lovely saltwater creeks, which provided calm waters for her and easy access for me. If she went to the actual beach, it was always with a friend. Elena loved the waves and delighted in them chasing her as they broke on the shore. I wasn't confident to even go in the shallow waves alone yet, fearful that if I was knocked down I would not be able to get back up and walk out.

On this particular day, that all changed. "Come on, honey. Grab your bucket and spade. We're off to the beach!" I declared cheerfully. Her delighted little face spoke for itself, as she rushed off to grab her things. The stroll from the car down to the beach through the soft sand was easily manageable. We set our things down and walked into the shallows.

Elena screamed in unhindered joy as waves came and lifted her up, all while she held on to my leg happily. As my toes dug into the moving sand below, water came and went. My feet and legs stood firm against the small waves. The nurturing energy of the ocean water washed gently back and forth against me. We were both playful and madly euphoric. What a joy "normal" can feel.

My feet were a little tired afterward while driving home, but certainly no more than a regular day of pain. I wondered how they would feel the next day, hoping they wouldn't be in increased pain from their efforts. They weren't. It was just back to a regular day of living with RA—tender and painful, but not crippling.

It didn't matter. That one single day of feeling normal again gave me a tiny glimpse of possibility. It also whispered a gentle reminder to never lose hope. Life could certainly change for the better. Sometimes it might be a long, gradual process. Sometimes it could happen in just one moment.

While remaining as present as possible, I certainly felt myself opening up to even more of those moments of possibility and positive change. I was ready to own my role of happiness, health, ease, abundance, and success.

It only takes a moment for a miracle.

41

Whether it was a pattern of life to stretch me, or whether it was an old part of myself hanging on for one last bout, I'd often been presented with an immense test between significant surges forward.

As I was enjoying some ease, consciously admitting that life *was* becoming easier, the calm slipped away overnight. Wrist pain woke me with a vengeance. For three days I was at the mercy of the disease, having to completely avoid driving and any other exertion on my hands. Such a level of physical pain naturally prompted emotional release. Feelings lingering in the background, waiting for the right time, came forth and out.

My medications were so hard-core that they usually took care of the worst of the pain. With the absence of most grains in my diet, time between flare-ups was extending. By halfway through the first day of the current flare-up, though, I had to lean on the painkillers. Sadness and despair had returned, but frustration was added to the mix. The lid on the bottle of painkillers was child-proof. What I most needed was under a lid that refused to open. It took every ounce of effort to break through the increased intensity of pain while tightening my grip to undo it. This was not the first time I had become exasperated by the impracticality of such designs.

The pills helped a little but not entirely. A fire raged. Every passing minute witnessed my balloon of faith and gratitude deflating a little more. It was a pinprick—not a huge burst, but a gradual, undeniable leak of all that had been sustaining me.

Throughout the whole journey with the disease and through my life, trusting in God's plan for me was usually one of my strengths. Not now. I was done with finding the blessings and allowed my anger and sadness to be expressed. Retrieving any-thing good to focus on or to sustain me was just not possible.

"I hate you, rheumatoid arthritis!" I cried at the disease. "I don't care how much you have taught me. You are still here and I *hate* you. Get the fuck out of my body. I hate you. *I hate you.*"

With the intensity of pain in my wrists equivalent to resting them on hot coals while a steamroller went over them back and forth, my heart bled out its tears. There was no boundary or con-trol left. I was so damn sick of being strong and positive, weary of finding the blessings. What blessings were there to be living in revolting physical pain consistently for years? It was fucked. I hated it and everything it robbed from me. In the quiet of night in the rainforest, I sobbed for all I had lost, especially life without pain.

Immense strength had been needed to constantly think past the disease, particularly when physical strength and pain-free liv-ing were so long ago. Too many future thoughts had compensa-tions to accommodate the disease. I didn't want them to, of course, but they often did. On very strong days, I dared to imagine life free and fully mobile again. On regular days, it was a consistent effort of mental discipline, emotional molding, faith, and spiritual reconnection to stay on top of it all—to stay believing in the pos-sibility of change.

On this occasion, my emotions and focus plummeted down-ward. The long-lost freedom of basing decisions on abilities drew heart-wrenching moans of grief. Depths far deeper than ever before were accessed through the release. Memories of my life with a strong physical body flooded back. I could feel myself walking with my confident, happy rhythm that only a lover of walking knows.

When I'd lived in cities—Sydney, Melbourne, Perth, London—walking was my main means of transport by choice. Sometimes I would leave home in the morning, simply to go walking. It was not unusual to arrive home at dusk, having had only a couple of half-hour stops in the day. The rest of the time had been spent in an easy stride, loving the discovery of things at ground level rather than through a window of motorized transport.

I missed that part of me intensely. Never before had I realized how much. I sobbed as numerous happy memories surfaced. How could it be that that part of me was gone? I had tried *so* hard to live an authentic, good-hearted life, embracing all the challenges that life sent me. I was so damn done with it now.

As well as walking simply for pleasure, it had often been my savior through challenges. Walking had been my loyal companion. Whenever I didn't know what else to do, having reached another point of surrender, it would accompany my thoughts. Together we made an amazing team, capable of solving almost any challenge I was going through. Off I'd go, allowing the rhythm and momentum to soothe my soul. It always did. Now I couldn't even do that.

Damn this life. How on earth could all this be for my highest good? Hadn't I burdened myself with enough penance for all the guilt and nonsense I once carried from others? Hadn't I reached a great enough level of self-love and kindness to now reap the rewards from my efforts? With my heart begging painfully for answers, tears continued to fall.

"For goodness' sake, God, I need a break. I need life *easy*. Please," I whispered in exhaustion. "Please help my life move forward now, into a new and easy chapter. Please, God. Please reconnect me to that part of myself that knows how to truly allow this through."

In such deep sadness, other memories surfaced, giving me further access to a deeper well of grief. Now I saw myself playing guitar and singing, enjoying laughter-filled times with friends, celebrating through music and song. I hadn't truly appreciated just how much I had loved sharing musically, in both giving and receiving tunes.

Initially my longing to be heard, to have my message reach people, had certainly been a strong driving force as a singer/songwriter. In those early days of my musical path, there had also been healing to do in my relationship with my father. He had given up his own music career by choice and stubbornness. As a result, he had not been hesitant in bullying me about trying to create such a path for myself. Yet my longing to be heard and express myself through song helped me stay focused, despite the cruelty he served up in those days.

As our relationship healed, he eventually became a supportive advocate and did his best to show interest. I can't say that I ever truly developed a yearning to share much with him, though. Perhaps the scars were just too deep. Also, his opinion, good or bad, no longer carried much weight for me. I had found my own approval instead. I felt happy for him that he had reached a place in himself where he could at least show a more supportive side.

Performing had also helped me become a much more open person. It played a very significant role in my healing at the time. Eventually I lost that unbalanced drive around my music—to be heard, to prove myself, to succeed. Instead I was able to be present, happy, and simply enjoy sharing my songs without fear of how they might be received or delivered.

Now my longing was purely for the love of music itself—for the love of *my* music, my songs. I remembered the ease of my fingers dancing on the strings, the complete presence and surrender when a new song was flowing through, and the euphoria that air in the lungs from singing offered. It all felt so easy and loose. Oh, how I longed to feel that freedom in my hands again. My voice also grieved the loss of its expression through that channel. My heart missed both its sound and the feeling of joy when singing along to my guitar.

That evening offered the deepest experience of grief I had known since being ill. The release was healthy. It also signaled a time for change. I was done with the hard life. Enough was enough. I had always tolerated and accepted challenges, perhaps too complacently or philosophically. But I was so damn done with it now.

I don't know how long I sat there in dim light, drained from my tears and the release of grief. Eventually the tears did slow, and my breath returned to a more peaceful rhythm.

With a deep sigh, I rose from the lounge and began turning off the lamps. There was nothing more I could do, on any level. It was in God's hands now. As exhaustion and sadness carried my tender feet off to bed, I turned off the final lamp and sank immediately into sleep.

Tomorrow was another day.

42

I t would be lovely to say that the following morning I bounced out of bed joyfully. In an ideal world, that would be the case. The exhaustion from my grieving, however, had left me drained and still functioning a little in a state of sadness. Or perhaps it wasn't even sadness; it was more like despondency.

"What is the point?" I asked myself. "What's the point of trying so hard, to focus, to follow guidance, when dreams don't come true anyway? What's the damn point?"

The timing had felt so right. Kitchen moments were becoming enjoyable again. Other than the recent flare-up, my health was improving. I felt I had grown into a place of readiness for the dream house, being more at ease with the idea of its beauty and comfort.

All the timing had been indicating perfection that things were about to fall into place. My energy had been full of excitement and confidence. Faith was strong. Things were not falling into place at all, though.

I was struggling to find a point in the whole test of faith I had signed myself up for. The despondency gave way to a haze of nothingness. There was no hopelessness anymore. Nor was there hope. There was *nothing*, other than a lot of deep sighs and emotional exhaustion.

It was what it was, with no fight in me. The natural ebb and flow of life simply reminded me of the importance to just be, to allow life to be whatever it would be in that moment. In doing so, the haze of nothing would be allowed to rise and disappear more naturally, without further turmoil. I didn't have the energy to do anything other than nothing, anyway.

Thankfully meditation continued to be a part of my life. Those moments in stillness were the much-needed reminder of something larger at work. Always there existed another part of myself, one at peace in stillness and in the perfection of the big picture. Through meditation, that part of myself was accessed. It was time to deepen my practice again, through more intentional effort at the beginning of each session. In doing so, dropping into stillness was almost immediate, removing everything else but peace. From this place, guidance flowed up and out.

Recently, I had allowed my happiness to become dependent on the dream coming true. Once again, I needed to let go of the "must" outcome and reclaim happiness regardless. It was time to put wisdom into action, best done through kindness to myself. The recent releases of anger, frustration, grief, and sadness had been definitely needed. These emotions have their place and are much better released than carried.

I had a choice on how long I wanted to wallow in them after their release. By remaining in that state, I would be wasting the precious gift of life unfolding and passing by. In those sadder or exhausted states I had asked, "What is the point?" The point is to try to enjoy life whatever the circumstances, *regardless* of them. It takes courage and determination. Mostly, though, it takes conscious choice to focus on more positive things, guaranteeing an elevation of emotions. I had to keep going as who I was in that moment.

The lessons I had been given would have been totally wasted if life and I had stayed the same. Although it sometimes felt as if life *had* stayed the same, it really hadn't. It was always moving forward and evolving.

The learning had brought me to such a place of kindness within. As much as I hated to admit it to myself when I was angry at life, I really would not have changed anything with how it had unfolded. The lessons had been given at a pace I could grow with and had certainly not been wasted. I was indeed changed for the better. Having the peace and confidence to be me without influence from others was the greatest gift of all.

To acknowledge my efforts and the levels of self-kindness I had learned, I continued to find things to do honoring my needs. A band I loved was to play at a music festival not far from us. As the date approached, so did my determination to see them. I purchased the ticket. I had delayed until that point, waiting to see how my health was. Thankfully I was returning to a good ride with it. But when I contacted the people who Elena loved to be with when I was out, no success was found. Everyone was busy.

During her first year, Elena had experienced a couple of music festivals with me when she fit into the carrier on my chest. They were precious memories, having my babe snugly attached while I listened to acoustic tunes. Her smell was pure and I often kissed her little head while she slept there.

With the past couple of years not being easy, I had avoided music festivals completely. Now Elena was a little older and not so inclined to take off without me, and my health had improved. So I decided we would just go to the festival together since there were no suitable babysitting options remaining. As it turned out, I had one of the best days ever.

There seems to be a groove that Elena and I fall into when in unfamiliar territory. It is a happy, synchronistic one. As we meandered around the market stalls, danced or sat at concerts, and blew bubbles to the clouds, life felt remarkably easy and joyous. It reminded me of the London trip a few years earlier, and other trips we'd done since. The different rhythm we shift into works perfectly.

At the festival we ran into friends here and there, as well as chatted with strangers. Mostly, though, it was just my darling daughter and I embracing all of the sounds, sights, and delights. As the stars guided us home that night, she slept while I enjoyed the peaceful drive. I realized that I'd had a better time with her than I had ever experienced at *any* festival. (And I had been to *a lot* of festivals.)

If I had not committed myself to going to the festival by buying the ticket just prior to seeking babysitters, perhaps I would not have gone, thinking it might have been too hard for me. Instead, I committed to my own enjoyment regardless and bought the ticket. As a result, I was blessed with a fun-filled, delightful day with my little girl. It was magical and just what I needed to return to a place of lightness.

Life would continue to unfold. There would always be choices on offer. I might or might not live in the house on the hill, but whatever happened, I was going to continue giving this existence my best. Life was now and I didn't want to wake up one day wishing I had appreciated more of it. There were always blessings to be found.

While all of this learning was going on, those seeds I had already planted were still germinating in the background, ready to sprout into perfection when the timing was magnificently right. They had been planted and well nurtured. They would indeed bloom into something beautiful.

My faith was at last restored. "Welcome back, old friend." I gently smiled at it. "It's so nice to feel your company again. I've missed you. Welcome back."

43

Regardless of my perceived acceptance of the situation, when the time finally came around to move, there was definite resistance. We were to get the keys to the villa on a Monday afternoon. By the Thursday night previous, I had still done nothing to prepare for the move except for packing up the cottage. I kept waiting for a signpost from life to say we didn't have to move into it at all.

By Friday, the last business day before the move, it was obvious I needed to face the reality of things. Much of the day was spent on the computer and phone, sorting out the removal and service connections for the new place. It was not a happy day.

That evening I realized how much anger and stress the day had created in my body. I didn't want to carry that energy into my new home, so I organized a massage the following day. It was *heaven* and allowed me to experience a sense of normality afterward. Things were fine. The move into the villa was happening and somehow it would all be fine. At the very least, it would be better than where we were living.

Sunday, the day following the massage, was a joyous one. I was as organized as I could be and my feet felt amazing. For the first time in a few years, I walked simply to enjoy a walk, not to go anywhere specific. With Elena, I walked for an hour, including down and up a short but very steep hill. Elena rode on my back for some of the time and we stopped for a few minutes here and there. Generally, it was an experience of ease.

In the evening I acknowledged that through all of the trial and error with my diet, testing what worked and what didn't, I seemed to be getting on the right track. I was feeling much better than I had for a very long time.

I decided to give the diet a fairer trial by cutting down my medication. I was a little nervous, but there was no denying the detrimental effect the pills were having on other parts of my health. Time would tell how the change would affect me. For now, I would trust in my decision as best as possible.

Meanwhile it was time to move. Drawing on experience, an old part of myself surfaced and simply went into moving mode. My belongings had been in storage for 15 months, but there was no real sentimentality or reminiscing in seeing them again. Almost unconsciously, I got on with unpacking.

Those first three days were especially hard work on my body. My feet throbbed. My hands resisted the loads. Yet in other ways, it also rose to the occasion. It felt fantastic to be physically active again. Although exhausted, old muscle memories were ignited.

When I sat on the lounge amongst boxes the first night in the place, though, there was no excitement or relief surfacing. The place just looked so white—white walls, white tiles, white blinds. Wondering if I would ever feel at home there, I tried to remain trusting beneath the exhaustion.

Unbeknownst to me, a subtle shift was already under way. Quietly it was gaining momentum. As the unpacking continued over the next few days, small moments of delight started seeping through, gently but surely. With each box unpacked, the home and I bonded more. It continued to whisper a loving welcome, which became more audible by the box. While out shopping on the fourth day, I realized I was actually looking forward to going "home."

The next two weeks unveiled many wonderful changes within. The increasing sense of home was glorious, particularly enhanced once the cupboards and fridge were full of healthy, divine food. My recipe books were out in full swing. Music played throughout the home, as Elena delighted in having her own room and her mum's renewed energy. We bought fresh flowers to strengthen the connection to home. I replaced all the white blinds with curtains of color.

All the while, Elena was fast becoming friends with other children in the complex. As our place was tucked away in a private little corner with no through road or passing traffic, the managers asked did I mind if the young children rode their bikes and scooters out front. I was more than happy to oblige. Many afternoons when the children came home from school, Elena was out playing with them on her scooter and bike. I could hear her from the villa, giggling, chasing them, and growing up quickly.

The day after moving in, I gifted myself with an automatic garage door. When it rained a couple of days later and we drove straight into the garage, which had an internal door to the home, I realized I had received exactly what I had asked for—ease. The home was not only comfortable. It was easy. For where I was at with my health, it truly was perfect.

Thinking about the big house on the hill, I could now acknowledge I wasn't actually ready for it yet. There was no sadness in this admission. The house was there. It was still for sale. But it was a big house to manage, something I saw I didn't actually want to do yet. Managing this small home was already enough. Some days, if my health was not great, it was almost too much.

There was much in favor of small homes. As a lover of simplicity and de-cluttering, I'd often seen the value of reduced belongings and commitments. The little villa, tucked away in a private, green corner of a small and friendly neighborhood, ticked so many boxes on my wish list. I had *never* imagined the home would become such a pleasant surprise.

Life had shown me just how much it knows our needs better than we sometimes do ourselves. As Elena slept and I sat in my new, gorgeous, colorful reading chair, I glanced up from my book, feeling the peace the dear little place was bringing me. While working at my desk, all I saw was greenery out the window. The backyard was a perfect, manageable size, which the building manager mowed for a ridiculously low fee whenever required.

The greatest joy was in the kitchen. When I had been in a very low chapter many years earlier living well below the poverty line, I'd taken a photo of my fridge contents. It had been *completely* empty except for one solitary jar of jam. Now I took a photo of my fridge in my own home, laden with organic vegetables and divine, healthy treats. It was a fabulous gauge on how far I'd come in many regards.

Within three weeks, I'd hosted a few friends for lunch on different occasions. I was completely in love with food preparation again. The ceremony of sharing returned to being a celebration. It was not only my mind that was happy. My body was too. In a short time it had become more upright. Its shape no longer said, "I sit down all of the time in pain."

As there were still physical challenges and progress to be made, I began to experience increased relief I wasn't in the big house on the hill. What this chapter offered me was a chance to recover, to bring myself back. To go from the pain and stagnation of before straight into a big home and large block of land would have been far too much.

Instead I was blessed with something I *could* manage enjoyably. This time would allow my abilities to increase more naturally, one gentle step at a time, without pressure. Too much physical exertion could have sent me backward. Managing this place wouldn't. When mopping the floor (the white, white, white floor), I was reminded I still did have some limitations. It was very hard work on my hands.

But in general, my body loved the increased activity when paced out a bit. It also loved the bathtub, which I successfully enjoyed a few nights after moving in. Getting in and out was easy enough, even if I was still dependent on my elbows for strength. That was okay. At least I could have a bath without trauma.

The little villa was revealing itself to indeed be a home of healing and happiness. How perfectly things had flowed once I finally gave up the resistance. A month earlier I had sat in absolute nothingness when thinking about living there. Now I was experiencing happiness, amazed by the perfection of how things had turned out after all.

44

Most of the time, my intuition spoke so clearly that there was absolutely no denying it. Other times, I tried to reason with it *just a little*. When I had recently felt nervous about reducing my medication and my gut had supported that feeling, indicating I should wait a little longer, my mind attempted to reason and won out.

Needless to say, the move was not a good one. Within two weeks of reducing them, my body clearly told me it was not the solution I was looking for. By the third week, I increased them back to the original dosage. The pain that radiated from my joints was awful, constant, and intense.

What the experiment did was to act as a gauge on my levels of self-care. No longer was I willing to settle for that level of pain and discomfort if I didn't need to. I intended to embrace every single day as enjoyably and comfortably as possible.

The healing path continued. Some days there were horrible flare-ups, when plans had to be surrendered. Other days were remarkably manageable. We began small walks around our new neighborhood. I had loved walking with my mum before I became ill. Now I was walking with my daughter—her little hand in mine, both of us chatting away, until she couldn't help but expel some of her excess energy by sprinting back and forth.

When we stopped at the playground, I would walk up and down some steps to the slide while Elena played. A noticeable improvement was that not only *could* I walk down steps, but I could also use one foot per step without holding on anymore. I was still a little cautious, but there was certainly a new sense of gratitude and freedom.

The greatest joy was movement itself—having the choice to move again without the pain being crippling. If I pushed myself by walking a little too far or too fast, then my body would soon tell me. On a couple of occasions, I was rendered seated the next day. It was all trial and error, feeling my way through each day as it dictated. There was no denying I was improving gradually, despite the recent result of reduced medication.

After some more flare-ups occurred, I was reignited to finding a solution. When life's signposts clearly indicated I contact a particular naturopath, cynicism surfaced. I had already spent so much time, money, dedication, and, more important, hope in that direction that I now resisted. It surprised me to feel jaded and cynical about a path I had once been completely committed to for decades.

Eventually my inner voice could not be silenced. It was still calling me to find the balance between the natural and scientific approaches. Each flare-up reminded me I had to keep going if I truly wanted to have my physical freedom returned to me and to be free of the toxic medications I was on.

A place of acceptance had been reached. Rather than feeling ripped off that I couldn't do everything I used to, I focused on what I was gaining in terms of improvement. Memories were still there, but now they helped rather than hindered.

I refused to bumble through unconsciously. By putting my learning into action, I continued to choose gratitude and presence. Every small improvement was magnificent. Focusing on that certainly helped ignite joy rather than loss. Thinking about damage or defeat just equaled lack, whereas wellness equaled abundance.

When I met the new naturopath, one of the first things I said was I needed a teacher. I was not looking for him to save me but to show me what I was missing on my body's path to healing. He was delighted and replied that teaching is all he *could* do for me anyway. I liked him instantly. He had also been a registered doctor in Australia and other countries but had given up with the bureaucracies of the Western medical system. Ayurvedic, Eastern, and other medicines were also a part of his wisdom and qualifications. All in all, he was a pretty amazing guy.

The first thing he did was start me on a three-week detox program to rid my tired body of anything draining its wellbeing.

We would move forward from there. Numerous tests were carried out, with him telling me things about my body that others had completely missed. One thing he did say as a result of those tests was that I actually had an incredibly strong body underneath the disease. It was our job to reconnect me with that.

My Feldenkrais teacher had said the same. Through those lessons I was slowly learning how to create a new organization within my body through awareness of movement. Whenever I'd had an hour session, I felt so much more normal. In fact, there were parts of me that felt *incredibly* normal for a while. It was inspiring. It helped me see that, effectively, I was really only ever an hour away from normal! If I could continue the learning, full health did not have to be years away. It still existed within me. I just had to reach a place within myself where the blocks to accessing it were removed consistently.

Each of us has a body that is a unique wonder of creativity. Despite their apparent similar structures and makeup, our healing journeys are an individual thing. While I removed or added further foods to my diet and tried this herb or that, there always seemed to be people who needed to share their opinion. Whenever I received well-intended though unsolicited advice telling me how I could be doing it better, what treatments would work best, or what spiritual practice would benefit me, I smiled gratefully and patiently.

None of my research had been wasted. It all formed a place in my learning and in wisdom gained, not through external sources but from life experience. I remained open to advice when I asked for it. It was just the advice beginning with "You should" that I was developing an aversion to. My new naturopath gave his advice in a respectful way, noting where I was already on my journey. He shaped his teachings around *my* body, not someone who has a particular disease. It was refreshing.

As the seasons changed and autumn departed, the balm of gentle winter sunshine nourished my gradual outdoor activities. I was so thankful to live where winter was manageable. Our new little home was warm compared with most other houses I'd lived in during winter. It continued to surprise me in the best ways.

My life was changing. It was telling a new story. It spoke of a woman who could find amazing blessings in her simple life. She no longer dwelled on hardship, pain, or who she used to be. She was a peaceful woman proud of who she already was and excited by who she would continue to become.

The old story no longer fit.

45

To assist creating a new story, I committed to stop speaking about the disease except when truly necessary. I had thought I wasn't speaking about it terribly often, preferring to focus on better things. When making the real commitment, however, I caught myself often saying snippets here and there. It was time to nip those in the bud.

I wasn't in denial. But it was just time to be speaking of only wellness when possible. It was time to move forward in new ways. Deciding to try more yoga, I questioned my readiness for a full group class. They had never really been my thing anyway—solo practice at home was more enjoyable for me—but it wasn't happening enough. Elena insisted on copying me for one or two positions, and then climbing all over me for the rest. So I booked some private classes, one-on-one with a teacher. The following week, the day before my first one, she had to cancel all the classes I had booked for the next month. I took it as a sign it was time to try a different direction for my recovery instead. Yoga classes could come again later.

Having been stagnant for a few years, the increasing strolls were lovely. My body was asleep and had been for too long. An area that truly needed awakening, to assist the recovery, was my lymphatic system. Feeling rather courageous, I took Elena to an indoor trampoline park. As she instantly jumped like crazy on her tramp, I began with gentle, tentative bounces on mine. I was concerned about the pain in my feet intensifying, but it remained the same. So I grew braver and finally after a few minutes, I fully jumped. It may not have been quite like the old days when I could jump to the ceiling, but who cared? I was jumping. We laughed and jumped for what seemed like ages. Jumping, jumping, jumping!

Celebrating how alive and amazing I felt afterward, Elena and I headed out for lunch at a beachside café. My energy was happy and light. Smiling from ear to ear all day, I knew I'd had a breakthrough. I was indeed moving forward and the trampoline was my ticket. The following week we headed back to the trampoline park and did it all again. It was just as wonderful. My body responded with delight. Blood and oxygen were pumping in a way that left me feeling more alive than I had in years. My energy was lighter and my limbs looser.

The benefit of the trampoline park was that we could each have our own trampoline. However, heading there only once a week and having to work it in with other plans and the schedule of the park would not work ongoing. So I ordered a trampoline online for our own backyard. We could still go to the trampoline park if we wanted sometimes. Sharing the tramp at home with Elena would at least be better than nothing at all. We could still take turns in having our own time on it, too.

That wonderful feeling from activity was the lure I needed to keep moving forward. Tasks I may not have been able to do for the past few years now didn't seem as daunting. Standing on a step to adjust a wall hanging, making beds with fitted sheets, carrying the washing outside to hang as a whole load instead of a few pieces at a time were all simple but significant changes. If I couldn't do other jobs when I tried, it was okay. What mattered was that at least I was now trying.

On another particularly beautiful day, the winter sun shone happily. Living where the winter is mild and summer is hot and humid means that in many ways, winter offers me much more freedom than summer. My fair skin loves winter. On this day, it was just too magnificent to stay indoors. Even though it was a scheduled workday with Elena being in care, I had to gift myself. Off to the beach I went.

I walked leisurely along the shoreline as gentle waves splashed my feet. The glorious sun nurtured my soul. It truly was a perfect day, so incredibly magical in temperature and atmosphere. A year earlier, walking on sand was completely impossible. Now I was walking on my own. It was heaven. After the walk, I sat in the shade of a tree, watching the soft waves lapping a pristine beach. The ocean was a remarkable blue and not a cloud could be seen above. Although the occasion was really only a few hours, it was like a lifetime of experiences. The gentle breeze kissed a contented face.

I was on a roll. New York, now only two months away, also felt more manageable. The fear associated with my capabilities whilst there was disintegrating. Rather than being concerned about being able to walk much and enjoy the city at that level, I was confident that enough ability to do so would be present. Excitement about my current life and my future was beginning to dominate rather than occur every now and then. I was the new me more than the old. A rebirth was well and truly under way.

When a financial statement arrived notifying me of a forthcoming payment I had been waiting on, it was well under what I had been expecting. In my state of presence and gratitude, I wasn't at all bothered or concerned. I just thought, *Okay*, and turned my thoughts into focusing on the blessing of even that amount. It was a good wake-up call to be respectful of the savings I did have remaining. There was still a home and life to support. It did mean, though, that my income was substantially under what I had thought it would be for the year. Having survived several years of poverty, I knew I would survive. No matter what, I was better off than I had been for all those years.

A couple of weeks later, I received a phone call telling me there had been a mistake on my statement. More money would be coming, an amount much more in line with my expectations. While researching apartments to rent for the New York trip, I knew the quality I wanted. Yet during those two weeks, until I heard I was receiving more money, I had started considering walk-up apartments. Staying in one of those would have added an extra burden to my energy and wellness.

When I realized I would be able to rent a decent apartment without stairs, an old part of me wondered if perhaps I could save that money and handle a walk-up. It was time to change my perspective.

Not only did I deserve to be comfortable; it was now time to actually celebrate my success. It had taken a couple of years to even truly *acknowledge* it to myself, finally feeling proud of what I had achieved. Now I was beyond acknowledging it. It was time to *celebrate*.

From the moment I'd received the publishing contract, I'd been consumed in motherhood and then chronic pain. Now I was breathing again, feeling lighter, and realizing what I had actually achieved through all my earlier years of resilience, focus, surrender, courage, and faith. If one way of celebrating was to rent a truly comfortable apartment in New York, then so be it.

Less than two months remained before the trip. I was doing great with my diet and thoughts. Life was feeling possible. There was really only one thing left to do to get my body prepared.

It was time to get jumping.

46

O nce the trampoline arrived, my body continued its resurgence to strength. Slowly but surely, daily changes were under way. My muscles, long asleep, gently awakened. The best part of all was the fun being had in the process. I continued to do what I could with patience, jumping most days.

In the meantime, further tests with the naturopath revealed the toxicity in my body was still higher than its energy. Until we tipped those scales, my body stood little chance of truly recovering. So further supplements were added to assist the continued detox, and it was off to do more colonic sessions.

The continuing deterioration of my oral and visual health was impossible to ignore. The conventional medications still continued to assist me in positive ways, but their toxicity was clearly not helping in others. Despite very recent dental work, a tooth flared up so badly it had to be removed. I hated losing it. Then another needed fixing a week later. Then to top it off, I came down with the worst flu I had *ever* known.

Here I was trying to focus on only wellness and it felt as though my body was falling apart. My calendar was filled with medical appointments of all kinds. Yet life was still helping by blessing me with increasing financial abundance to cover it all.

The money I was expecting was late. This actually worked to my benefit as the Australian dollar was falling and the money coming was in a foreign currency. Every day the pending amount increased. I took this as a deliberate blessing from God and from the part of myself that had finally stepped up in self-worth. I also took it as a sign to support the things that mattered most to my wellbeing—comfort and ease.

To honor that blessing and those needs, I finally booked an apartment for New York before the dollar fell further. It was beautiful, comfortable-looking, and on a high floor of an elevator building. It was also next door to a grocery store with a wide range of organic food. The boxes for both comfort and ease were ticked.

When the overseas payment eventually arrived, because of the altered exchange rate, it had increased the perfect amount. It was almost the exact difference between the cost of the walk-up apartment I had been considering and the comfortable one I actually rented. Effectively, life had supported my courage in honoring my needs by paying the difference for me.

I felt like God was saying, "Don't think at all about money now. We've got that covered. You just focus on your wellness." Sometimes it had been the other way around. I had health, but was doing my biggest learning through my relationship with money. Or I had a decent love relationship, but was learning through job dissatisfaction. Whatever lesson I most needed, life gave it to me through the perfect channel for that moment. Right now I felt true flow with money for the first time in my life, but my body was continuing to offer the biggest learning.

Food continued to be a fabulous teacher. Illness had brought me to a level of self-love where organic food and truly healthy eating were now normal to me. It no longer required an effort or justification. Even when I was well, I knew I would continue eating this way.

Just as a full fruit bowl had once been the measure of feeling rich when I was living in poverty, food continued to mean so much more to me than just something to put in my mouth. It represented self-love, abundance, and wisdom. It encompassed all my life.

Still, my body was exhausted, stressed by so many appointments and the demands of solo parenting. Being the only adult in our little family was an honor *and* a challenge, especially to my own wellbeing and balance. But overall, I was proud of myself for where we were at, for the job I was doing as a mother, artist, businesswoman, and individual.

Meditation kept me connected to a place of peace each day and beyond. But it wasn't quite enough. My energy was truly shattered and heading further downward, especially when the flu took full hold. Coughing tired me out, often leaving me with a headache. Everything left me beat. Each new appointment scheduled, supposedly for wellness, just added stress.

One morning, I woke up choking, unable to catch a full breath at all. I rushed to the bathroom and held on to the sink for support, hoping the standing position would help. Gasping for breath, over and over, I watched my face turn red and tears flow involuntarily from my eyes. Reaching for a full breath while choking, coughing, and heaving, my thoughts rushed to my darling girl, who was lying in bed, watching me via the en suite mirror. She had seen me sick with the flu for a few weeks, so didn't grasp the severity of the incident, thank goodness. I *had* to find my breath—if not for me, for her. Finally, *finally*, I managed a small burp that seemed to unblock the airflow. It took a little while longer before I felt truly safe again.

When breathing returned to a more manageable place, I sat on the side of the bed as little Elena sat up and hugged me. We held each other for ages in silence. It was obvious I needed help. I was not well and needed a break. So that day I postponed what I could. Elena and I spent most of the day playing peacefully at home, doing puzzles, reading books, and watching *Frozen* for the millionth time. The only trip we took was a quick drive to an organic juice shop, as I had no energy to make any myself despite now owning a new juicer my hands could usually manage.

During that same day, I spoke with my dear mum, as I did most days. In the evening, she phoned back to say she had cleared her calendar and was coming up for a few days to help out. I'd received many blessings in my life, but never had I felt so grateful as I did in that moment. At last, there was some light at the end of the tunnel. Once off the phone, I let my tears flow from overwhelming relief.

In order to take some time out from focusing on illness, that night I also booked a beachside apartment a few hours north. I needed a weekend away. We would head up there about a week after Mum's visit. I needed to step out of my current reality of sickness and have some good old-fashioned, wholesome enjoyment.

My body was teaching me significantly, including the importance of laughter and ease. It was up to me to make whatever daily choices I could to support lightness in my life, even when it seemed the furthest thing away.

Comfort, ease, *lightness,* and *laughter*—they were the words I was falling in love with every day. The more I thought about them, the more my emotions followed to experience them. This was where life was heading. I refused to believe anything else. Some of the best antidotes were coming to assist me: time with Mum, some days free of medical appointments, the healing winter sun, and the nurturing energy of the magnificent ocean.

Nature and love had healed me before. They would again.

47

Since moving into the villa, Elena had been delighted with her new room. Within a couple of days of living there, deciding that she was now a big girl, she had declared that she would be sleeping in her own room. My intention with co-sleeping had always been for her to decide when she was ready.

For the past few months, Elena had happily gone to sleep in her own room. I would lie beside her and read a story each night. Once the light was turned off, we would each make up a story about whatever subject the other suggested. They were our favorite times, cuddled up and whispering imaginative tales to each other in the darkness. Then she would climb on top of me and lie there until she fell asleep, at which time I rolled her off gently and tiptoed out of her room. Sometimes I would lie there longer just enjoying the feel of her asleep on my body, knowing that our evening ritual would change before long as she grew heavier.

Luckily, I now had the best of both worlds. My own sleep was finally settling into a better routine by having some solitude. I was also blessed to wake to Elena's little face and voice because she still came to my bed in the early hours. In my sleep, I would hear the patter of her feet coming down the hallway rug. In she would climb, teddy tucked under her arm, and snuggle into me. Then we'd both return to sleep. It was a beautiful routine.

My sleep had been terribly shattered through motherhood and RA. I still dealt with pain in my body every night, particularly in my hands, whilst trying to find comfort through sleep. Those hours before Elena came to my bed at least allowed me to retrieve longer stints of solid sleep, moving from three hours at a time to even five hours some nights.

As soon as Grandma arrived, the routine changed. At the insistence of a determined three-year-old, I was banished to Elena's bed so she and my mother could sleep together in mine. It was nice to let go, though my role with my mum was changing as she was now older. A part of me was going into care mode, hoping *she* was getting a good night's sleep. She told me she was and I could see she delighted enormously in the special time with her grand-daughter, but I still thought she looked a little tired each morning.

Together Mum and Elena decided she was going to go home with Mum for a few days to visit her cousins. That possibility had not even crossed my mind, but once the words were spoken, my body ached in relief. For the following three days, it was just me. As a parent, you can dream of all the things you would do if you had the time. I certainly had. Now my body just insisted on rest. There would be no achieving this or that, going here or there. It was all about gentleness. To ensure I honored this, the skies opened. Winter rain fell solidly for three days straight, supporting my retreat.

With no responsibilities and amazingly no appointments, I could move slowly or not at all. Making a huge pot of soup was a great move on the first day, sustaining me throughout. My ribs were delicate and in extreme pain every time I coughed. What was obvious, above all else, was just how lacking in quality sleep I had been for more than three years. Exhaustion was a large part of my problem.

Knowing there were no responsibilities at all waiting for me upon waking, my body finally let go into sleep properly. For three nights I slept at least six hours before stirring, only to roll over into further sleep. It was heaven, particularly with warm flannelette sheets, a big quilt, and rain pouring down outside in the darkness.

I knew I was ill and tired, but I hadn't realized how desperately I'd needed the help that came. When it did and I felt the pressure release from my body, I was able to view life more clearly again, renewed for another chapter.

With those few days of Mum's visit followed by the few days in solitude, I discovered a beautiful sanctuary within, full of magic and possibility. I walked out of them in wonder and delight, feeling lighter than I had in a very long time. The eyes of the child within saw everything afresh. Although it was only a matter of days, the rejuvenation experienced felt like I'd been away for a couple of weeks.

I was especially reminded of how desperately I needed solid, good-quality sleep. That had to be my biggest commitment to my body. I had the diet quite mastered. I was doing more exercise, including jumping when I was well enough. Fresh air was a part of my lifestyle. And when possible, I absorbed the healing power of gentle winter sunshine.

As I fell into a deep sleep that last night, hugely looking forward to being with my little girl again the next day, I sent out a prayer of thanks. It wasn't just for the opportunity to sleep as well as I had. It was for the reminder of just how much God loves us and wants us to be happy.

Help is always there. Sometimes we just have to ask or acknowledge the need first.

48

Three winters previous had been the trip from my home region to the coast where I'd had the epiphany that we needed to live in a coastal and warmer region. A friend had supported me as I tried to walk on the sand, gently helping me sit on a rock while I watched her and Elena play. It was bittersweet and ripped my heart out since I couldn't play with my little girl.

The following winter the same friend had supported me onto a sand dune so I could at least see and smell the ocean again.

The next winter, she held my elbow for support as I walked onto the sand. She also carried a fold-up chair so I could sit near the water.

This winter, during the trip further up the coast, she offered no assistance since none was needed. She simply walked beside me as a friend and then relaxed as Elena and I played in the shallow waves. After some time, I joined her sitting on the beach, while we covered Elena in sand at her own request. It was a fabulous gauge of how far I'd come and a stark reminder of where I'd been.

The time away turned out to be a wonderful antidote. In particular, it offered time with that dear friend and another who lived locally. Their love and support were the best medicine. Winter sunshine also put on its absolute best face, with not a cloud in the sky. Elena likewise loved the discovery of new playgrounds and time at a different beach.

On returning home, the flu eventually lost its hold and began easing up. A second session of colonic treatments ended. Medical appointments seemed to ease off a little. Our social life continued to be satisfying and without so many other time commitments, I was able to enjoy it more. We had made good friends in a short time. Two women in particular, both older mums like me, both with little girls around Elena's age, were becoming more and more like family every time we connected. Our girls all played wonderfully together, while us mums could let go for a while and simply enjoy our friendship.

Everything was changing, for the better. That descent, along with the recent sabbatical of rest and time out, had brought me back to a whole new level. I had to go down to go further up, as often happens in life just before a new surge onward. The cloud was lifting and instead of me coming out where I entered it, I came out further along, above it.

My body felt the strongest it had in three years. My spirit was lighter. Work opportunities, aligned with random desires, flowed almost as quickly as I imagined them. Invitations to global speaking events also increased. With improved mobility, it was now possible to consider them. Thoughts of broadening my world again provided hope for a continued return to wellness.

Elena and I were in a great space together. My willingness to honor my own needs by continuing to create space in our plans could now be enjoyed. We continued to have people over for lunch. Being able to enjoy the kitchen and express my love by providing nourishing meals to friends and little ones felt great. It also left me feeling normal instead of craving something that was not. And there were some wonderful days with no plans at all. Elena often led the way at those times.

As I returned to jumping on the trampoline once more, everything felt easier. My health and strength were undeniably improving. Each jump was higher or a little more confident. Every jumping session was a little longer. The aftereffects were less noticeable in my feet. Everything felt much more possible again.

Each lesson I was given was perfect for where I was. The more I could embrace this, the smoother my journey was. As I dared to honor my greatest potential, I was still asked to do the work, to face my fears. That was actually the joy of it. I stripped away all that held me back from my truest calling. Not only was this living an authentic life; it brought great joy. By expanding myself, over and over, stretching to become who life was asking me to be, I ventured into unknown yet familiar territory.

It was the land of my heart's roots, where I belonged, even if I had no conscious memory of being there. The calling grew louder. Occasionally the voices of fear or distraction muffled it. It remained waiting during such times, only to congratulate me when I returned by placing me further along the path than when I had left. My heart never stopped calling me forward and the more I allowed it to be heard, the quicker its pace.

There was no denying I was experiencing a new momentum and that I was stronger emotionally. Upper limits I had once feared now felt simple. Some of the previous fears even felt somewhat ridiculous. When I thought about all of the rationalizing and turmoil I had worked through when imagining living in the house on the hill, I could feel only compassion for my old self. To live in such comfort and beauty would now feel perfectly acceptable and natural.

The guilt or shame I had previously experienced when imagining earning a substantial wage was also long gone. Millions of people in the world still earned much more money than I did. I certainly wasn't in the league of those folks yet. But I was also no longer in the league of poverty, a state and story that had been familiar to me for much of my adult life. I had grown comfortable with the idea of earning good money and allowing myself the wellbeing and choices that flowed from that. It really didn't matter what anyone else was earning anyway. My own perception of abundance had improved, which was what was needed for my own flow.

So it was with complete faith and a quiet excitement that I continued to step forward. Whatever was coming was fine with me. I was on the right track and life was teaching me just how perfectly it presents its love to us.

49

While we enjoyed the little home we had bought, it was still not the dream one. I was peaceful for what it was—a perfect place for life at the moment, a gentle stepping-stone. The privacy and space I dreamed of did not yet exist, but many other positive characteristics did. On a global scale, I was still a very blessed woman. A dear daughter, a darling mother, food, shelter, clean water, work I loved, friendships, and relatively good health were all mine.

In this more settled space, I came to reflect quite differently on the previous decades of roaming and relocating. Back then, a part of me did know that I was running from pain. When I finally stopped and honored the desire to settle, I slid into that very dark period of depression. The pain had caught up with me. As raw as that chapter was, stripping me bare of my past, it was also an enormous gift of growth.

It allowed me to then move forward more as my true self, less restricted by the opinions of others. Those changes became a part of me, rather than just some brilliant insight, realized then forgotten. This continually helped strengthen the permission I needed to live in a more balanced and gentle way, free of caring how I would be perceived.

Being so much more settled now, I also realized I hadn't been running from only pain. I had been running from my own potential, which is what actually awaits beyond pain.

My present dream was to stay in one house, in my true home, and grow from there. There was no need to run anymore. My love of travel and discovering new cultures still existed, but it was free of restlessness. It was now just a thirst for learning and adventure. Home was where my heart was.

I wanted to plant a seedling and watch it bloom into a fully grown tree, strong in its roots, broad in its branches, solid in its magnificence. I wanted to watch Elena grow up with that tree. I also wanted to measure my own growth, my own ability to bloom, through it. I wanted to stand strong in my roots, at ease with my natural growth, flexible to bend with life, and magnificent in my own sense of self. I wanted to bloom into my absolute best potential, and allow that vision to continue expanding in its own natural way.

Thoughts of the grand home on the hill still lingered. Without the pressure of an unhappy home environment, they were much more peaceful and accepting. We drove past it about once a month, instead of weekly. It had been taken off the market for the time being, but the owners were still open to offers. I began to wonder for the first time since meeting it whether the house really was the home we were destined for.

It felt good to question myself. The dream of home still existed. I hadn't actually seen the qualities I loved in any other house, but I was surrendering control and opening to the possibility. It was a nice feeling. I still loved the house on the hill completely. I just wasn't so fixated and rigid about the outcome anymore.

In the meantime, my thoughts about winning the lottery had also changed immensely. Some weeks went by when I didn't even bother buying a ticket. We had a nice little home. I'd also finally grown into enjoying the feeling of earning. As my income flow had increased, particularly from many seeds planted in previous years, I began to enjoy the sense of achievement it brought. Just as I had learned to experience the healing of my health one step at a time, I liked watching my abundance increase in the same way. Knowing I created each step through my work and the conscious choices and action I had made felt empowering. Supporting Elena and myself in such a way was bringing unexpected pleasure.

There were times, many actually, when I found playing the roles of both parents quite hard—being the nurturer *and* the provider, the good guy *and* the bad guy, the feminine *and* the masculine. It was a constant juggling act, but I seemed to be doing it pretty well. Elena continued to be a remarkable child, full of wisdom and grounding. I reassured myself I was actually doing a great job, proud that I was providing for her well: spiritually, emotionally, physically, *and* financially.

Although I still purchased a lottery ticket occasionally, it was certainly not in any regular fashion anymore. Even then, it was possibly more out of habit than hope, with the practice slipping further away all the time.

To honor my father, I had added number 26 to my ticket when he died since he had been so adamant it would come up. Mum had been doing the same. It took 10 months after the dear old man passed away before the number was drawn. I won about $80 and Mum about $100. We both thanked Dad and laughed that we could now stop playing the lottery at last.

Immediately following that incident, I realized just how shaped by the lottery and my father's habit of it I'd been. It was a genuine relief to not have the expectation of winning in the background of my mind anymore, for it not to be the only solution or possibility. I could now let life be what it was, without that hope always lingering, controlling how abundance should flow to me. I didn't have enough money yet to buy my dream home, but when the timing and readiness were right, I would—and it would come through whatever source it chose.

I didn't need enough to live off forever right now. Money was energy, a constant stream that would keep flowing. I didn't need a deposit like water contained within a wall of a dam—stored in excess, not allowing flow in or out. Needing it all right now was just fear based, connected to the possibility of running out. I didn't need stagnant energy attached to my money. Enough for now was enough, and I had that comfortably.

With my addiction to simplicity and a love of culling my belongings, I might have been overwhelmed with too much money too soon anyway. Like my clothes, I would have just given away the surplus. With my winning-the-lottery dream having many fine details after so many years of shaping, I had often imagined such scenarios of helping certain people out. But I didn't actually *have* to buy every friend a house or be the channel for his or her money to come through. I could pass kindness forward and even help out a little financially when possible, but I didn't need to save people anymore. Each of us has our own lessons with money. It was not up to me to find the solution for every person I loved.

More and more I liked the idea of earning and growing into my dream. I didn't want to land somewhere before I was truly ready. By growing into increased finances, I was able to adjust and enjoy my sense of achievement. Coming from such low levels of self-worth and poverty, any increase felt great. I didn't want to miss the ride.

By allowing the energy of money to flow, it also pushed me past complacency or fear and made me rise to my potential. That is what life was revealing most to me through these years of illness and the conscious choices I now made on a daily basis: As much as we might want a quick fix, when we do experience the sense of progress and the achievement of overcoming challenges, we actually step into our best potential. In that place reside joy and the opportunity for incredible happiness.

50

The trip to New York was finally upon us. As the city limits came into view from the plane, a sense of achievement seeped through my jet-lagged exhaustion. *I did it*, I thought. *I really did it.*

Memories surfaced of when I first began researching my interests for New York. It had been while living on a farm, just coming through the haze of depression. I was still dependent on food vouchers from charity organizations back then. So traveling anywhere, let alone to New York, was way off my radar of possibilities at the time. Yet I planted a seed and nurtured it with imagination and faith for five or six years, until I saw the city come into reality before my eyes.

The pace and excitement of New York swept us all immediately into her embrace. We felt compelled to be out and about, caught up in the thrill of the city's heartbeat. It wasn't until three days there that I realized I was actually in a state of complete exhaustion. Unable to sleep at all while sitting up in the plane, my body had been ravaged from the trip.

The hum of traffic and air-conditioning units, added to the sirens from the fire and police stations within a block of our apartment, just added to the challenges of the quality sleep I now longed for. With my immune system suppressed, another flu took hold. The polluted city air flooded my exhausted body. Delirium took over.

I recalled once reading how sleep deprivation is a form of torture used to get prisoners to talk. I could understand why they would surrender—I would have done almost anything for some quality sleep. Earplugs didn't work. The flu raged on, I coughed constantly, the subway stifled me, and I seriously questioned why my heart had called me to this city with such intense longing.

I thought of home, our sweet little place of peace. It was obvious that we not only lived in one of the most incredibly beautiful countries in the world; we lived in one of the most beautiful regions within that country. People holidayed to our region all the time for a reason. It was heaven. Yet here I was in New York City, having paid a small fortune for the apartment and trip, longing for the clean air and ease of home.

Having Mel with us was indeed a treat, though. With time to roam while Elena and Mel went off and did their own thing, it was wonderful. On other occasions, the three of us had outings together. Just having that extra support with parenting made it so much easier, particularly as I was *still* exhausted a week into the trip. The flu was not letting up despite my sleep improving slightly each night. Elena and I also enjoyed some slow, easy, special times, hanging out just the two of us. She was such a fabulous little traveler and I loved seeing life through her eyes.

Central Park and Riverside Park were both within easy walking distance. The moment I spent some quality time at Central Park, a sense of normality returned. It took being amongst such extreme contrasts to see just *how much* nature actually kept me balanced and restored. It was absolute necessary for my wellbeing. With clarity I understood I had to live in the rhythm of nature again. My own body and life cycle depended on it.

I had thought my heart had called me to New York to enjoy the excitement, food accessibility, and mixed cultures. The experiences of the past few years had certainly left me craving the excitement the city offered. But things were different now. With increases in global speaking invitations, the new life unfolding would easily satisfy my love of cities and a variety of cultures. I liked a little bit of everything and was creating a life that would give me that. I didn't belong in city life full-time. New York reminded me of that.

For the first time since discovering the house on the hill, my thoughts turned to living back in nature again instead. While that beautiful home had accessibility, privacy, incredible views, and space, it also had traffic noise. It was in a sleepy cul-de-sac but very close to the highway. That noise would only increase over time. I could get used to it. But as I fell asleep to the sound of traffic those first weeks in New York, my longing for falling asleep to nature intensified. I was grateful to know the difference between city sounds and nature at its purest.

Another thing New York taught me was just how amazing the food was back home. I had to travel and source the food I wanted, but it was accessible enough. Even in New York, while organic food outlets were more common, I still had to find them when out and about. They were not on every street corner. Until organic food was mainstream, it would always require some amount of effort, no matter where I lived. Our home region had strong organic influences already. It was time I appreciated that fact more rather than wishing I didn't have to travel a few miles to find what I needed.

As these insights revealed themselves, I allowed more fluidity into my dreams. It was with quiet excitement that I wondered where my true home actually lay. Just knowing it would be back in a country setting brought a feeling of pleasure and curiosity. It seemed the house on the hill was actually waiting for someone else. In the meantime, a beautiful home was also sitting quietly somewhere, surrounded by nature, waiting especially for us.

Isolation would not be a problem anymore. That had been a state of mind, through illness and necessary healing. I was enjoying an active social life again and this would continue, wherever I lived.

Each time I went out for a day on my own in New York, another wave of gratitude hit me. I was *walking*! As a means of transport, for hours, I was doing it the way I had dreamed. The difference from how it used to be was that I walked slower, meandering happily. Illness had taught me how to stroll. It became symbolic for how I was living all my life, strolling rather than pacing with pressure and overexertion. So stroll I did, stopping whenever necessary, for a rest and a moment of stillness and observation.

The novelty of walking down steps without holding the railing never left, with a reminder every time I descended to another subway platform. Although the flu lingered, my sleep improved, along with my increasing appreciation and enjoyment of the great city we were in.

It was a good choice to be there for as long as we were. We had time to slip into a groove in our own way. Our mornings were slow. Mel enjoyed time out with her new church friends. She and I each enjoyed individual nights out for concerts and Broadway shows. Other nights the two of us enjoyed long conversations in the apartment once Elena was asleep. A huge pot of memories was filling, each becoming more positive by the day.

I thanked my heart for leading me to New York, even if the reasons for it had turned out to be much different than anticipated. I thanked God for giving me the courage to honor my heart and for the insights I had discovered about my true needs for well-being. I thanked New York for the role it played, for the turning point it became.

As I learned to fall asleep to the wail of sirens and the hum of traffic, my heart also knew there would come a time I would fall asleep to the lullabies of frogs. The house on the hill had become ingrained in me. I had felt myself living there for so long that it needed a wake-up call for me to let go.

I surrendered with trust. New York actually set me free.

51

When we arrived in New York, it had been just over a year that I had been taking the conventional medications. They had reached their plateau of obvious improvements six months earlier. The only noticeable changes in more recent times had been once I started working with the new naturopath.

Having mobility back was the first noticeable sign of their help, and one that brought immense pleasure. Even if I had to soak in the bath at the end of a long day's walking, at least I had been able to walk the distances I was. I could stroll several blocks of the city, gently, before needing to rest. Each day's walking created an unintentional tour of juice bars as they were the rest stops my heart and map led me to. On most occasions, if I thought of somewhere specific to go, walking there was considered as a possibility.

Not long before the New York trip, I had picked up my guitar again. It brought tears of joy to discover I could now hold three chords with my left hand. As I had to hold the formations differently because of the inflexibility of some fingers, it looked as if I was sticking my finger up at anyone sitting in front of me. The fingers on my right hand wanted to dance again, too, as their own memories awakened. Their flexibility was still restricted, so a slow process of rehabilitation began.

Just being able to sing along to basic strumming was heaven. My wrists weren't strong enough to put a capo on the neck of the guitar to offer a variety of tones, so it was pretty much just those three chords to start with, and only for a few minutes at a time. At least I was playing slightly. I could do a simplified version of a love song I once knew. Thoughts of Jeff surfaced as I sang, reconnecting me to that dream.

It had been quite some months since we'd seen each other. Although romance had been absent from my mainstream consciousness for a while, my feelings for him remained unchanged. In fact, I was getting a bit tired of being patient and surrendering. Through pain and fear in my past, I'd become a master of disguise. I'd not given Jeff even the slightest inclination I had feelings beyond friendship. It was time I started facing those fears upon my return.

Lugging my guitar to New York had not been an option owing to the lingering disabilities in my hands. I figured I would be fine for the time we'd be away. Playing had not become such an obsession or need again as it once had been. Or so I thought. As I walked past a guitar store one day in Midtown Manhattan, my feet turned on demand, taking me straight inside.

All the acoustic guitars were in a sealed room. As I entered, the smell of wood and the sight of the magnificent instruments overwhelmed me. I tried to fight back tears of grief, but they won. My heart ached with incredible sadness. There was no point getting a guitar down off the wall. The frustration of immobility in my fingers was too much as the wave of heartache continued.

How could it be that I couldn't play properly anymore? Why did something I loved so much have to be taken from me?

I knew the answers to those questions. The disease had brought me gifts like nothing else could have. Even the inability to play had made me appreciate my music on a whole new level. Oh, how I longed to play properly again, though. It was killing me.

There was no way to go but forward. So there and then, I purchased a little travel guitar, one that I *could* carry easily, and one that would at least allow me to muck about regularly, no matter where I was in the world.

Each day in New York, I played for a little while until pain ended the session. Like the walking, playing was reconnecting me with an old part of myself. It was reigniting the memories needed to call me back. As the sirens echoed below our 26th-floor apartment and the hum of traffic never ceased, my ears tuned it all out. All that existed were the tunes that flowed through me. The more I focused on that reconnection, the more hopeful I became.

I simply had to get out of the way and allow life to flow. That was all it wanted from me. My greatest show of appreciation to this gift of life was to enjoy it as best as I could, whatever the circumstances.

Life would always lead the way. It would again call me to serve, but in a way that was wholesome for my own soul's journey too. In its own miraculous way, it could bring about the very best of circumstances to benefit all. This would all flow even more easily as I allowed more enjoyment in.

To trust, surrender, and accept my own potential was my calling. It could take many acts of self-kindness, conscious choices, and immense courage. I was human, after all, so fear was a part of the process of growing into my readiness. With that vulnerability also came power. Rather than be scared by my potential, I could continue to embrace it. With one gentle step at a time, I would grow into that readiness, aided through every conscious decision I made along the way.

52

As the flu took hold of my body at the start of the New York trip, it was clear the conventional medications had served their purpose. They had helped return me to the level of mobility where I was now. It was at least somewhere I felt I could improve upon, a little less aided from here. This was a place where memories and feelings were blending, pulling me forward. The walker was now walking more on her own.

The medications continued to suppress my immune system, leaving me repeatedly vulnerable to other illness, including the flu. I wanted my body back, including the fortitude it once showed against virus.

Thoughts of reducing the medications did not evoke quite the depth of fear they had six months earlier. This time I had spoken with the rheumatologist about my intention. It made him shudder in disbelief, but he politely educated me on the hypothetical situation of one reducing their medications, and which order to do it in. There was much to consider.

To the rhythm of my walking during the New York holiday, my thoughts regularly contemplated God and the ability of divine intelligence to reverse the disease and its symptoms. The source that made my heart beat without the help of my conscious mind was the same source capable of healing my dear body of disease. The divine intelligence that showed my body how to grow Elena in my womb still existed in me. God, who guided my body into creation, was still and always a part of me. This place of infinite wisdom and love existed everywhere, including within my own body.

I could improve my diet, return to exercise, take supplements to assist my restoration to wellness, meditate in a state of peace, and visualize all I liked. All of these had their important place on my journey of self-kindness and healing, hence why I continued to do them. So was the case with consciously enjoying my life.

The very best thing I could truly do was to acknowledge the divinity within myself and stay as connected to that as possible. My consciousness of this, *recalling* this connection, *was* my connection.

If ever there was a time of surrender, this was it. Physically and mentally, I had applied myself to the journey as the most devoted student. My focus could no longer be on finding a solution. The best thing I could do to honor my soul's connection and purpose, was to just be and to remember there was something so much more powerful and capable within me already at work.

Shifts happened faster all the time. The way my walking had improved and speaking opportunities had flowed, it was clear. I just had to allow it. The stronger my experience of oneness became, the easier my needs and desires were flowing. I simply had to *be*. The state of allowing I had been taught now revealed amazing ease by manifesting in other areas of my life. It was just as possible for it to do so with my health, providing I didn't block it with unnecessary thoughts.

Imagining becoming well was obviously much easier to do when I was actually improving. It helped reawaken memories from old parts of myself. The things that carried me through most, though, were my faith and the belief that God and divine intelligence were on my side.

The more awareness I developed during conscious day-to-day thought of the divine healing happening within, the more power both my conscious *and* unconscious minds then gave it. In order to train the unconscious mind, where all seeds of manifestation sprout from, I first had to sow and nurture them constantly in the conscious mind. Simply *remembering* divine intelligence gave it permission to weave its magic. The more often I consciously recalled this, the more easily its healing work could be revealed. It was a new height of wellness I began aspiring to.

As I walked the streets of New York, listened to a bird singing in Central Park, or was lulled by the swish of the shoreline on the Hudson River, my thoughts returned to the spiritual healing already going on within me. On one particular day, they were brought back to something that had occurred only a week before we flew to New York.

I had attended an event held by my publisher. Dr. Wayne Dyer and Anita Moorjani were holding a workshop called "I Am Light." Wayne had been a wonderful advocate for my work, speaking of it onstage in recent years. As well as being inspired by these two wise, beautiful people, I had the blessing of meeting with them. Wayne had interviewed me on his radio show about a year earlier, so our connection was in place. It was wonderful to finally give him a hug of thanks.

Just over a week into our New York trip, Wayne, who had just returned home to Maui, left his body, passing away. It was an unbelievable loss and shock to all who loved him and his teachings. I felt incredibly grateful to have spent time in his physical company so recently, including sharing a lovely conversation and that long-overdue hug. During his workshop, I had made some notes of insights I was having. One was actually how much more I had needed to focus on divine intelligence doing its work.

Back in the New York apartment, Elena, being an author's daughter, was "working" by writing a book on my computer. She typed away happily in her abstract form. As I wrestled between determination and fear of reducing the medications again, allowing spirit to do the rest, something stopped my mental debate in its tracks: The recording of my interview with Wayne Dyer started suddenly playing on the computer.

I asked Elena what she had pressed, but she assured me she had stuck to the alphabet keys. As she had often written books on my computer, I believed her. I went into the program where the sound file was kept, but it was jammed, refusing to be switched off.

Dear Wayne. He was insistent on continuing his role as a teacher, even beyond this earth. I sat myself down to listen to the interview and to his beautiful voice flowing through. I recalled the insights I'd had during his workshop and how I had just let my focus slip into fear rather than into connection.

I couldn't stop smiling all day. God was talking to me through Wayne, in a way that ensured I would listen. From that moment onward, my conscious thoughts of the divine intelligence within my body started becoming more and more natural and increasingly a part of my unconscious thinking.

Instead of trying to find solutions for my health, I was in a place of *complete* trust. As my fitness improved with each step on New York streets and my heart lifted with the freedom of holidays and the power of faith, that simple phrase *Let go, let God* sounded like pretty fine advice to me.

53

I t was difficult to believe and a little hard to accept that our time in New York was coming to a close. It felt as though we had been there for five months, not five weeks. As the holiday drew into its closing week, a mixture of happy anticipation for home and a love of New York danced around each other.

The city, which had completely overwhelmed me physically, emotionally, and mentally in that first week, had drawn me into her crazy magic. I had sourced my favorite food outlets and learned to catch buses more than trains. I had even given tourists directions. I loved the city and could easily understand why she drew so many people into her arms.

During my last free evening, I stood alone at a crossroad watching the flow of people. The city lights were enticing us all to stay out later. I could even feel nostalgic about the traffic. Well, almost. I wanted to freeze that moment in time for *just* a little longer. Earlier that day I had spoken at a writers' workshop. The hours of freedom wandering the streets for one last time were a perfect closure to a positive day.

The city had changed me. Even the clothes I bought represented a new me, the one I had been evolving into. I was more comfortable with better-quality clothing. A certain quirkiness was still attractive as I was always, at heart, an artist of sorts. My tastes had been changing for some time, though, and New York opened my eyes to broader styles. Visions for my work were also inspired and formulated. I had grown into myself and felt courage building to back myself more. Plans formulated to employ an assistant. It would only be the first step of many toward building my team. I stepped up to new levels in accepting my professional role. I had a message to share and it would not be honoring my life if I did not step up and share it well. New York had helped me own and fit that vision.

Numerous memories of laughter and joy had also been created. The happiest moments of all were when I felt Elena's little hand in mine as we went off on our adventures. The changes in her were impossible to ignore. She was reading street signs, telling me which way to go on the subways although I already knew, ordering her own food at shop counters, and as always, choosing her own clothes in shops and for daily outings. New York fashion had clearly affected her, as she donned random accessories and her new love-heart-shaped sunglasses with whatever blend of floral, stripes, stars, and rainbows she could find.

I loved that she found elements of nature along the concrete footpaths. It could take a long time to walk even one block at times as we investigated the colors on fallen leaves, an acorn, an interesting stick, or whatever else her eye was drawn to in the natural world.

Of all my outings with Elena, going to a particular spot in Riverside Park were my favorites. The journeys there were adventures in themselves, but sitting on rocks by the water was where they always ended. All of the busyness of the city fell away behind us, over the rise, out of sight, out of mind. While we sat in the shade, the breeze off the Hudson River was refreshingly calming. Sitting on the rocks for ages, we'd tell tales of mermaids and other very important things.

I proceeded with the reduction in medication. Initially, noticeable signs of doing so were increased inflammation and pain. Yet there was also a sense of relief, to be free of the side effects of that particular pill. My vision felt clearer almost immediately. Regular lethargy also lightened.

Despite my efforts to focus on wellness and divinity over the previous three and a half years since being diagnosed with RA, it felt different this time. The commitment came from a deeper place of resilience. Recent increased movement allowed me to connect with the feeling of wellness as a better fit rather than just an imagined ideal.

The more I focused on divine intelligence, the stronger my belief in healing grew. It was not a blind faith. It was a commitment to conscious action, conscious focus. It was not only divine intelligence being contemplated. *That* I could accept with ease. It existed with or without my focus, even though I was increasing my awareness of it for the intention of healing. What was more difficult to accept was that divine intelligence was actually divine love.

Realizing the enormity of love that existed within me and learning to connect with that was painful and somewhat terrifying. Allowing myself to receive such unconditional and infinite love was more than my human heart could comprehend. It took immense courage to even contemplate my worth on this level as it represented me in my most unlimited greatness, as it does us all. That level of love resided within me, as me. It was already there, but in my humanness, the thought of being so lovable, to receive such unconditional love into my conscious heart, was bewildering.

Accepting that I was loved infinitely brought tears to my eyes. Although a part of me could certainly rationalize that I deserved that love, another part of me was still learning how to accept it. This unrestricted love from the divine infiniteness of God was always there. It was mine simply for existing and waited only on my readiness.

Allowing *so* much love through, learning to *truly* receive it, left me like a fragile little girl who had wanted love so much, but had learned that it was too painful. Now life was asking me to be brave and open up to the immensity of its purest form—as divinity within me and everywhere. It did this through the lure of glimpses into my potential and the increasingly audible call of my heart. I was being pulled forward with a longing to know and experience this level of self despite how much it scared me.

The incident with Wayne reminded me of how infinite love is. He continued to love his students and teach them because he was one with divine love. I was a part of that, too. During decades of meditation, I had often reached states of such intense love and bliss that I had sobbed with the enormity of it all. At other moments of complete presence in nature, I had felt the infiniteness of divine love. So it was not an entirely new feeling.

What *was* new was my effort to connect with it in my day-to-day living, *well beyond* the levels of awareness, gratitude, and love that I usually did. New thought patterns were being called into creation so it would be me in my every-state as I went through regular life.

Life was asking me to open up to the absolute fullness of love that it wanted to share, to incorporate into my new and more ready self. It was beautiful, incredible, and certainly overwhelming. I was being asked to be an example of infinite love in the most constant, conscious state of being as I could be.

We are all asked this, in one way or another. Our heart calls us to this potential with every yearning it shares. I wanted to be brave enough to experience my own divine potential in my every-day being, to *know* that infiniteness, not just flick in and out of it during inspired moments.

I spent quiet reflective time in communication with my cells, letting them know that the other cells some of them were attacking were actually love too, and that it was safe now. I didn't need to attack myself. I needed only to love. Continuing to meditate on divine love encompassed me with gentleness.

Clearly, some walls were being pulled down. The finite concepts of love, shaped by a scared little girl who decided that love was pain, were dissolving. The overwhelming beauty of my spiritual self was crossing into my physical self in a way like never before.

A blending, a new expression of my divinity through myself as a woman and person, was unfolding. Although there was intensity in the realization of what was actually happening, and some enormous fear of accepting such infiniteness, it was some of the most beautiful learning I had ever done.

This pull, to rise up and be the best we can be, is something we all share. We truly are one. And that one is love.

54

I did actually love the disease. I didn't love *having* it, but I did love it for who it had made me. The love was genuine, real, and quite overwhelming when I realized its actual existence. No longer was there resistance. Instead there was a total trust in the perfection of it, accompanied by a deep faith that more freedom of health was to unfold.

In that first week or two of the reduced medications during the New York trip, old pain did flare up. It was a grungy sort of bone pain, threatening its full potential. Although I was still living with pain every day, sometimes it did not warrant too much attention. It was just there, but not disabling in the way it once was. The recent increase reminded me how severe and debilitating the disease could be.

I chose to continue rising above it, knowing that the medications were not the long-term solution. It reminded me of a long time back when I had been a heavy cigarette smoker. When I was truly ready and it came time to quit, any time I wanted to give in to the addiction, I would ask myself, "If not now, then when?" I knew I had to ride out the challenge or I would never move forward. That question helped me endure the internal battle, ensuring I left that habit of self-hate behind forever in my late 20s.

As I worked toward the reduction of medications and increased wellness, I again asked, "If not now, then when?" I endured the increased pain, continuing to focus on my cells loving one another, on me loving my body, of divine intelligence speaking perfectly to my whole biological system, and especially of divine love flooding through me effortlessly and with unblocked flow.

On the second to last day in New York, I had been walking up a hill on a tree-lined street of brownstone homes. It was a glorious day, mild and sunny. As I walked, I felt a muscle in my thighs working my legs, a muscle that had been dormant for the duration of the disease. It was fantastic to feel it come alive again. I was not strolling up the hill. I was striding, something I had always loved to do on an upward slope. Another shift had also occurred: I was not limping at all.

The last day in New York was spent with Elena and Mel in Prospect Park. There were many other activities we could have done, but we simply had an easy and memorable day wandering the park, stopping at playgrounds, watching the swans, and just being. Mel headed out in the evening. After Elena and I had enjoyed a fun bath time together and she slept, I sat in my pajamas, reading. I was in a state of complete contentment. As our trip home began the next morning, the comprehension of changes that had unfolded for me in New York was gratifying.

Although the limp was still sometimes there in weeks following, it was losing its prominence. The more I called on the learning I had done through the Feldenkrais sessions, the less I limped. With a focus on my hips being the center of gravity and a determination to not walk too fast, hence not leaning my body forward onto sensitive feet, walking continued to improve.

The trick to longevity and endurance with walking was to go gently and steadily. With each piece of improvement, it was clear it was not going to be a spontaneous remission. Rather, what was unfolding was a gradual reversal of the disease and its symptoms. In a way, it was much nicer as I could then witness the changes at a noticeable pace, not that I wouldn't have actually refused a spontaneous remission.

The grungy pain that had surfaced upon stopping the first pill had gone. It was just regular pain again, no different than when I was on the drug. As it continued to level out, my body grew even stronger. Although there were still moments of surrender to the disease, more of my physical freedoms continued to be awakened. Subtle yet powerful improvements were under way.

One day soon after, while home in Australia, I dropped my keys in a parking lot. They fell underneath the side of my car. In a flash, an elderly lady was there, down on her knees, laughing as she reached under my car and retrieved them for me. She was a gorgeous, spirited being, and as I thanked her, I caught a flash of myself in her. It felt great imagining being so nimble and having a believable vision to aspire to.

My story had changed. I was happy to speak of wellness and improvement. The identity of a sick person had served its purpose and given me a reasonable excuse for time-out and other permissions. Self-love, and the results from those lessons through illness, were ingrained enough now for continued acts of kindness to myself.

55

As each of the medications I was on took six weeks to show full effect, I also gave the recent reduction the same time. Gauging it after that time was a joy. I was no different, no worse for not taking it. The inflammation had leveled out to its lowest level so far, but I still couldn't play guitar well at all. Nor could I run, but I could function independently, undistracted by the presence of any severe pain. Some moments limping existed. Some not. It didn't matter. A life of expanding choices was being given back to me through the freedom of increasing movement.

Two months after that reduction, I decided to approach the next tier. At that time, two weekly pills remained, the immunity suppressants. These were also the hard-core toxic ones, bringing the most benefit and damage simultaneously. As I reduced the intake, it felt fabulous knowing there was less toxicity going into my beloved body. I would wait another six weeks until I judged the results properly.

Things were looking up, though. There was no denying it. Applying lotion or oil to my body had been quite difficult until then and at times, even impossible. No matter how gently I applied it, the pressure on my wrists was just too painful. I did what I could sporadically. After those two reductions, I could happily return the habit to my daily routine. The difference this time was that as I did so, I told my body how much I loved it. Sometimes my thoughts were simply, *I love you*, as I applied the lotion. Mostly though, it was, *It's okay—I love you*. My body, my dear friend, pulsed with gratitude.

In the meantime, I was tiring of focusing on recovery rather than normality and wellness. Four weeks after returning from New York, I had a short trip to Austria to speak at an event. This time Elena stayed with her grandmother while her aunts took days off work to spend quality time with her. She rode horses, col-lected eggs, gardened, swam, chased cousins, rode on her uncle's shoulders, and experienced a fun-filled time during my absence.

The joys of modern technology kept us connected daily. I did miss her dearly, particularly after we saw each other's faces and talked online. And each time I saw a mother with a young girl, my heart ached in pain. Yet I enjoyed the time away, simply having no responsibilities other than work, which I also loved.

Without the old levels of debilitating pain, I was enjoying more presence with my work again, allowing me to experience my heart's expansion in that area. For a long time, I had done only what I could to keep my business floating along, little more. Now as my physical strength improved, mental clarity resurfaced, further aiding my enjoyment and readiness for further growth in my career.

Like all women who are artists and mothers, or all people who love their work, I would probably always live with a divided heart. It was the pull of motherhood and loving my child against the pull of the independent, creative self. It was a choice I had made when opening myself up to motherhood, and as much as the divided heart definitely existed, I would not have changed a thing. Elena was the greatest joy I had ever known. Being her mother helped me daily to become my very best self.

Even so, having some solitary time was a healthy blessing after recent burnouts, illness, unbalance, and feeling overwhelmed. Reconnecting with more travel was fantastic, too, particularly since I honored the needs of my body for comfort this time by not traveling economy class. The effects of the long-haul trip to New York with its non-existence of comfort or sleep had been too much trauma on my body. It was an important wake-up call. Comfort was not only a desire. It was a necessity.

There were a couple of days in Austria when my health chal-lenged me, but overall it was an enormously positive time. I loved revisiting Europe after more than a decade. Throughout the time, I adhered to all the protocols of my naturopath, which included three different drinks of supplements spaced out each day at specific intervals. It was a pain in the butt, going out and about with three different bottles in addition to morning and evening supplements.

During the actual flights, I couldn't take fluids on board because of quantity restrictions by the airline. On the flight home, I realized how wonderful and normal it was to not be focusing on any of it. Despite my best efforts to focus on wellness, when you are tethered to a clock and medications, it is a constant reminder of illness.

It was time to step away from the conscious effort of healing and to just be. I had been led further toward the Ayurvedic path and learned about gentleness in a way I liked. As well as encouraging gentle eating for my gut, its teachings included making decisions that added ease and gentleness to my life in general. It offered freedom from the rigidity of the other dietary dogma I had experimented with. There was loving flexibility within its philosophies and guidance.

It was springtime—a new season in nature and a new season in my life, and time to build my team to create more balance. Things had become busy again, much more than I enjoyed. I had to honor my need for ease through both comfort and balance. Comfort was sorted. Balance needed more attention.

The first step was to employ a cleaner. Although she came for only two hours a week, the gift it gave me was astonishing. I realized how much time and effort I had put into the house, just to stay on top of things. It was the only way I had coped when I was so frail and disabled. I would not have been well enough to ever catch up again. It wasn't perfection I was aiming for, just a sense of management. As a result of that habit, I was still working far more than I needed to maintain our home. Those two hours employing a fit and happy woman to clean was like having a fairy godmother come through with a magical feather duster.

A couple of times, I arranged more care for Elena to avoid future burnouts. Employing a personal assistant in addition to my current virtual assistant was also on my mind. I needed to train someone for more of the business side of my work so I could enjoy more time on the creative. I was an artist first and foremost, and the yearning to honor that could no longer be ignored. I wanted to get offline.

The call for home persisted but was no longer distracting. During those weeks in New York when I realized my need of living in nature, a particular town a little further south began standing out as a suitable possibility. I needed to return to the bush, where no sound of traffic at all existed. Even when we'd been in the hot shed hidden in the rainforest, we could still hear the highway traffic a couple of miles away.

There was nowhere in the shire we were living where we could have both silence and easy access to fresh, organic takeaway food. My diet would always be a priority from now on, but so would the choice to not have to prepare our food every single day. As I hadn't attracted a food-loving assistant yet, I at least needed to live near organic cafés. This little town offered that, as well as a great homeschooling network, easy access to the tribe of wonderful women I belonged to, and accessibility to most else I needed for ease and comfort.

As travel was increasing with several trips overseas already booked for the following two years for both work and family holidays, it was clear that my love of cities could be satisfied during those times.

Accepting that the original house on the hill was not actually our future home, I briefly returned to the real-estate pages online. It exhausted me instantly, so I ceased, but not before noticing one particularly gorgeous place. It was only a 10-minute drive from the town in mind and was coming up for auction soon, meaning there were open houses happening. I went to check one out.

On exiting the car, my first thought was, *All I can hear is the breeze.* I took a deep breath of the clean, mountain air. Birds' voices joined the song of the wind. That was all there was, nothing but a perfect symphony of nature. The location was heaven: ocean views, privacy, a separate studio perfect for a homeschooling community, separate guest accommodation, and 40 acres of rainforest. The home itself was lovely, spacious with lots of light and views. I didn't have the funds to buy it, but I had the trust that if it were to be our home, the funds would come in time.

The auction occurred while I was away in Austria. By the time it came around, I had completely surrendered to whatever would happen and forgot about it entirely. It was not until the next morning that I realized the auction would have happened, and obviously, I was not a part of it. I later learned of its sale through a friend who knew the original owner.

There was no sadness, only gratitude. That home had shown me there were other houses out there that would also suit my desires. The feelings I longed for within my home had been planted and were leading me to where I was supposed to be. Not one ounce of doubt existed in this regard. Our house was waiting and it would include everything I had come to love through my search for home.

56

Settling back into life after the two trips away, I couldn't deny it anymore. It was time to deal with my feelings for Jeff. The experiences associated with the home search had increased my faith and confidence. They were direct reminders that the feelings I yearned for might still come, but in a different form from what I had envisioned. This reasoning was still working in regard to my thoughts of Jeff, too. If he was not the right partner for my soul's evolution and joy, then the feelings I yearned for were coming through a partnership with someone else. I told myself it was fine however things turned out between me and Jeff.

When I made the decision to phone him and share what was going on inside me, it was not all actually fine. I was like a nervous teenager with sickening butterflies and intense fear. It was awful. I delayed calling until some conscious breathing returned me to a calmer state. I had hoped it would feel natural and joyous, as our friendship always had. Still the nerves persisted. Courageously, I dialed his number, sort of hoping he wouldn't be there. He answered in his usual welcoming, warm tone, delighted to hear from me and to reconnect. It helped me slip back into the easy dynamic of our friendship.

We caught up on his life first. After all, I was in no hurry to talk about myself. As the conversation unfolded, my gentle heart began to quietly break. It became clear Jeff's focus was elsewhere. As his friend I sat and listened, all the while praying for strength. His voice continued to share, but something in me moved out of the scene. A veil of numbness washed over me as his words became muffled sounds. I tried to be the best friend and listener I could be but wanted so desperately to just get off the phone as quickly as possible. Life then blessed me. Our call was disconnected midsentence.

As he is a busy man who does a lot of business by phone, this was not the first time his phone had gone flat during one of our conversations. Over the years, I'd come to know that if he was able, he'd go and plug his phone in and call me straight back. I hoped he wasn't able to. As I sat on the lounge absorbing what he'd shared, I prayed for help to surrender my feelings for him, for courage to still trust in the dream of love, and for the maturity to still be his friend. When it became obvious that he couldn't call straight back, I was relieved.

I wanted so much to cry, to let go, but felt too numb. How could I be wrong on this, too? How could someone else be the right person for me when it was our history that had left me feeling safe to love him, specifically him? How could I ever communicate in the way I did with him, with someone new? I yearned to curl up in a ball and sob, but I stared at nothing instead.

Jeff did call back later, but I chose not to answer the phone. Elena and I were having a beautiful time together in that moment. I didn't need to sacrifice a happy experience for a sad one. Later I wondered if I could even be his friend anymore, or at least, for the time being. It all felt too raw.

The thing is, Jeff was in a relationship. He had been for a long time. For much of that I had listened as a friend to the consistent problems that existed within it. I respected the emotional maturity of him and his partner as they had chipped away at things. Until that day before my father died, when I'd realized my feelings for him, I'd never seen Jeff as anything other than a male friend— a dear one, but just a friend regardless. I would have never imagined my feelings would change.

On that day I began to see him as the man he now was. The person he had become was talking about the potential of being single again, of facing the fact he had given his best but was still not where he wanted to be. He and his partner had already discussed the possibility of separating.

So it was not only my own fears that had stopped me sharing my feelings with him. It was respect for his and his partner's relationship. I hated that I had feelings for another woman's man. It was awful and something I battled with a lot. But as our conversations deepened even more over recent times, there was no denying a change in our friendship. We were much closer.

In the end, I did return his call, if only to get it out of the way. As the conversation unfolded, it was clear there was no choice but to be his mate and respect whatever choices he was making. Above all else, I did love him dearly as my friend. I couldn't turn that off. We laughed and talked philosophy as we always eventually did. He then steered the conversation back to my life.

Instead of being brave and telling him everything, which would have only flowed through tears of heartbreak, I spoke in third person. There was a man I had feelings for, I told him, whose focus was elsewhere, and I was feeling very raw and not at all strong in that particular moment.

I didn't say, "It is you, Jeff. I have feelings for you. I want to know you on every level. I want to know your soul and create a love that surpasses even our own dreams." I felt as if I was letting myself down enormously through the lack of this expression.

He was the same beautiful friend he'd always been, offering words of encouragement. That kindness made my heart break a little more, but by the time we said good-bye, I was happy to have connected with my friend again.

In the days following, I prayed for guidance. Mostly I prayed for the ability to surrender my feelings, to love him regardless of my desired outcome. I needed to set myself free, to be able to love him but not long for him, to respect his choice, and trust that someone more suitable was looking for me.

Through living in my dream of being with Jeff, I had lifted my expectations to a different quality of partner. I had grown used to the idea of emotional maturity within a relationship. The whole journey had increased my readiness for an incredibly beautiful relationship, free of the usual turmoil I used to attract. So even though Jeff didn't know it, he had already played a vital part in the realization of my dream for soul love.

I drew on faith to trust in the big picture. The love I yearned for was coming. It would just be in a different form, or at least a different person than I had imagined. That was what I believed in moments of strength. Most of the time, though, I allowed myself to feel all my feelings as naturally as they arose, often as heart-ache. Hope had obviously been carrying me through. There was nothing to buoy me up anymore.

I was weary of celebrating my womanhood on my own or through the sisterhood of friends. I needed to express myself within a partnership, with a gorgeous hunk of masculinity. Never in my life had I ever felt as ready for a relationship as I finally did.

At least one of my wishes came true. I could finally cry.

57

I t was time to set myself free. For too long I had carried those feelings for Jeff. If I was truly going to attract the right partner, I needed a ritual to intentionally release him from my heart and mind. So I wrote a letter, one that would never be seen by him but was initially to him. The more I wrote, the more the tears flowed, and the more other frustrations surfaced. Somewhere along the way, it became a prayer instead.

"Please, God," I ended up writing, "help me surrender this dear man to his truest path, without me losing any more energy or heartache to it. Please give me the courage to let go, to truly let go, and the faith to know that all is well, that somehow I will make sense of this in peace and gratitude, regardless of the outcome. Give me the courage to hand this over to you, fully and honestly. I'm so tired. I don't know what else to do. Please tell me."

When I was emptied, emotionally exhausted, I took the letter outside to burn. Memories of when I could collect my own wood from fallen branches and light a roaring fire under starlight came flooding back. Having released things this way before, I was aware of the power from such a ritual. But it wasn't like the old days. I didn't live in the bush anymore. On this particular evening, not wanting the neighbors to call the fire brigade or for anyone to interrupt my private ceremony, I simply set the letter alight and watched it burn its own fire. Staring into the flame, a sense of release followed. My prayers had been heard.

I wondered if Jeff would truly find the happiness he was seeking within his existing relationship. Would his partner either? But it wasn't my business anymore. My focus had to remain on the feeling of a soul partnership entering my life. If their relationship had already come to a natural close, then I would have felt differently. But in that moment of surrender through the flames, I had to trust that if we truly were meant to be, life would bring us together later. I wanted a man who was *available*, anyway, which Jeff was not.

I continued to tell myself the next day that I had told him enough. It was the right thing to do considering his situation. Yet the regret of not having spoken my truth began growing in unavoidable strength. There would be no denying its force forever. Life was insisting the words be spoken. We would either move forward as friends or say good-bye in loving peace.

The morning after the letter writing and burning ceremony, my health took a turn for the worse. At first I thought it was a flare-up from something I ate and that the worst pain would pass in a day, then reduce further over a few days. But the intensity of pain had not let up *at all* the second day. One of my worst fears surfaced: that the reduction in medication was not working and I would be stuck on the toxic pills forever.

The level of pain that surfaced took me back two years. I could hardly hold a toothbrush. Typing was out, so was dressing independently. The frown of pain returned to my face. My body stooped. Patience disappeared. Hope was extinguished. The recent feelings of normality were almost forgotten, while I carried my hands instead of using them.

It scared me how severe and sudden the downturn was. It was unbearable enough in the moment, but would absolutely crush me emotionally, once and for all, if ongoing. I couldn't allow myself to believe that, but was incredibly frightened. Two days earlier I'd been jumping and laughing on a visit to the trampoline park with Elena, full of physical confidence. Twenty-four hours later the pain was so intense I could hardly even recall the feeling of wellness. It felt that far away.

The emotional stress I'd been living with was causing as much damage to my body as any imbalance or physical strain could do. Stress was clearly a part of my life that needed more attention. Elena was sleeping much better, meaning I was too. Many nights I even had a full night's sleep while she slept right through in her own bed. But it was enormously clear my body's immunity was utterly exhausted by my emotional self. The severity of the recent physical pain was perfectly parallel to my emotional state from dealing with the heartache.

Three days later I awoke with ongoing debilitating, horrific pain. For the first time in ages I reached for a painkiller. As I waited for its effects to kick in, I curled into a tight ball on my bed and allowed the tears to flow. It was a scorching, humid morning. No energy for physical exertion or inner strength remained. I was absolutely shattered.

I yearned for more adult company and conversation. I yearned for love and support. It helped to admit my wounds. I could focus on blessings as much as possible, but sometimes I just had to allow myself to cry.

Dear little Elena came looking for me. She found me curled up and asked what was wrong. I sat up, drying my tears, and told her how frustrated I was with a disease in my body and that it was hurting a lot. She lived with RA in me every day. It wasn't like the disease was news to her. She accommodated my pained hands often in our movements together.

Honest expression had always been encouraged in our home. I didn't want her to see me cry every time. She didn't need that burden. But understanding that crying sometimes is a part of life was healthy knowledge.

After listening to my reply, she climbed on the bed and hugged me, saying nothing at first, just holding me. Then her little hand reached up to my chin and turned my face toward hers. With eyes of wisdom looking straight into me, she said, "Now listen here. One day that disease is going to leave your body and it's *never* going to come back. Alright?"

Bless her darling soul. I may have been in pain, but I did have much to be grateful for—my amazing daughter especially.

As the painkiller kicked in, the day began to feel more manageable. "Pack your bag," I said with a smile. "We're off to the creek." I watched her instantly transform back into a little girl again—excited, present, uninhibited, and free.

58

After loading our picnic stuff into the car, Elena climbed in with her swimming gear. It was time to change the direction of the day from the trauma of pain to a potentially happy occasion. The trip to meet up with other homeschooling families was heaven. As we drove about an hour into a lush valley, powerful escarpments hung over the farms and rainforests below. It was breathtakingly beautiful. The red-toned rocks of the cliffs were a perfect contrast to the green canopy of bushland. A brilliant cloudless sky allowed the earth's colors to radiate at their best.

I mentioned to Elena that I thought we might be heading somewhere near an old friend's house. I hadn't seen Bek for 16 years, since I'd first left the region. Yet every year at Christmas, a joyfully handcrafted card still arrived from her. Although we only had that annual contact, she meant the world to me. Recently we had reconnected and were trying to arrange a meet-up, but with her work shifts and our own commitments, it had not yet proven successful.

The further we drove into the valley, the more commanding the return to nature was. There was no denying the earth was calling me home. Everything made sense here, where an infinite well of peace was accessible and waiting. It was hard to believe the morning had begun with me curled up in a ball sobbing. Now everything just fell away.

The day was spent with about 20 adults and children. Swimming in a pristine water hole shaded by massive trees, we all connected with ease and joy. I loved watching my little girl learn from the bigger kids as they demonstrated how to use a rope swing. She was delighted and eagerly waited her turn, time and again.

I asked the event organizer if she knew Bek and her partner and if we were near Bek's house. It turned out they were on the very same property. We had driven past their home to get to the water hole.

These days, most people text or pre-arrange meet-ups. Not everyone is familiar with spontaneity anymore. This was an old friend, though, and there was no mobile phone reception to text. Surely we could just drop in? As we drove past the house on the way out, we heard some building noise. At least it was obvious that someone was home. I parked the car outside their fence with quiet excitement.

We trod gently up the stairs to the lovely wooden home, hoping to not be intruding. Elena jingled the old bell on the handle of the open door. A moment later Bek came into view and the warmest smile appeared on her face as she realized who was at the door. Walking down the hallway toward us with arms outstretched, delightful laughter burst forth.

We chatted nonstop over glasses of iced tea, followed by a tour of her home and two acres of heaven. As an artist, her flair was delightful with so many colors. Choices of plants in her garden were based on scents, shapes, and textures. Nothing was incidental yet it flowed with such natural ease it lifted us effortlessly. While I chatted with her partner, Bek chased Elena around their property, playing hide-and-seek. Driving home a couple of hours later, smiles of gratitude kept bubbling out.

We arrived back to our villa happy but weary from the hot day out and all of the swimming. After finishing off a large serving of watermelon together, Elena and I pottered about doing our own things in the home for a while. Then the phone rang.

Looking at the name on the screen, my heart instantly began thumping out of my chest. It was Jeff. Did I answer it or not? On the drive home, a song by Mary Gauthier had played. A line had stood out, as if I had never heard it before. "Truth always saves me when there's nowhere else to go." I had immediately replayed the song to hear it once more.

The same line came to mind loud and clear. There was indeed nowhere else to go but to the truth. "Tell him," my heart demanded. "Tell him." Looking down at the phone as it continued to ring, I sighed and finally answered, accepting the next step. I could not live with the regret of not speaking the truth any longer, regardless of how hard it was going to be. I had to trust that in the big picture, it was the right thing to do.

We chatted for a while about day-to-day stuff, though I have no idea what was really said. I couldn't hear anything over my beating heart. Finally, not being able to stand it any longer, I spoke.

"Jeff, you know the guy I was telling you about, the one I had feelings for?"

"Yes, Bron," he replied in a patient, gentle tone.

"It's you. I have feelings for you, Jeff. I wish I didn't, but I do. And I'm so damn tired of carrying them."

They were out. At last, the words were spoken. It was astounding how easily and naturally they actually flowed once allowed their release. Jeff told me he had wondered if I was speaking about him in that previous phone call but didn't want to assume.

Everything I had thought I needed to say had already been said in the recent letter. It had been released in the flames. All of those conversations I'd had with him in my head over the previous year were irrelevant. So now, I spoke with wonderfully enjoyable ease of whatever truth surfaced in the moment. Being honest with Jeff supported a habit I liked, the courage of vulnerability.

Eventually, on such a roll and unable to stop, I also told him of the lessons through the house—how I had thought I had found the perfect house for me, but it had only been there to help me grow into feeling more comfortable with something better. I explained how I considered that he may not be the right person for me, but how my feelings for him had helped me raise my expectations in the type of partner I now sought. Working through those feelings, I had already shed layers of fear that no longer belonged.

Thanking him for his unconscious role in that, we were both able to laugh again. It was our beautiful, safe friendship at its best. I told him how I respected his relationship and was simply sharing what had to be. It was with trust that I felt our friendship would evolve past these lessons.

Jeff had quite a bit to say, including things he admired in me. He also spoke of his situation, and while he and his partner were still together, they'd had some mutual time apart to think about their relationship. Listening, I realized that the things I admired in him were the reasons they were still together: commitment, loyalty, and integrity. I loved their endurance and despite my lingering heartache, I didn't actually want to see him and his partner separate. I wanted to cheer on their ability to grow through to the other side of their challenges. Their commitment and emotional maturity were inspiring.

It was ease and gratitude that concluded our phone call. The insights and surrender had been so powerful I knew I'd be okay, no matter what. A soul love was indeed coming my way. My courage to speak the truth had left me with an immense feeling of calm—one that almost felt foreign yet like an old friend at the same time.

When I fell asleep that night, it was with renewed peace and lightness. Immense gratitude washed over me as I was released into one of the best night's sleep I'd had in a very long time. The following morning, on coming out of my meditation, I noticed a distinct shift in the pain of my wrists. It had lessened considerably.

Jeff called in to visit a few weeks later and it was obvious our friendship had survived. We were closer but clear in our roles as friends. A week or so later I found myself driving behind him down a village street. I had recently bought a new car so he didn't recognize me. I could have phoned Jeff to let him know I was following. He would have stopped but there was no need. I felt peaceful to see him going about his day. As Jeff turned into a different street I sent him love and drove on, grateful at the perfection of it all.

Although it felt strange to have an open heart and no one to think about, I welcomed the adjustment. There was no conflict about wanting another woman's man or fear regarding the survival of our friendship. Jeff had played the role he was meant to. He had reminded me of the love that was truly possible between two committed people. He had helped me grow into a place of readiness.

59

Each day brought small but noticeable improvement to my pain levels. My first gauge was usually by how disrupting the pain was. In those worst moments, I had considered resuming the full level of medications. But confidence had returned to keep going in the direction I was, to see myself completely free of pills. With only one weekly tablet remaining, I decided to wait a little longer before the next reduction. I preferred to dwell in wellness rather than rush in prematurely. I was already moving in the right direction, so it was okay.

Life felt easier now, much more spacious in a healthy way. Simplicity remained an ongoing theme and was not a fixed point. Shaping my life by the day-to-day decisions made consciously, it was always there. Much had fallen away that no longer served. Life felt flowing and manageable, and not surprisingly, quite wonderful.

Stopping and looking back in reflection became an essential gauge of kindness to myself. With things flowing well, it was almost easy to forget new limitations or where I had been. It could have been easy to load myself up with more pressure and unrealistic expectations. Even though I was managing much better than I had in the four years of living with RA and being a solo parent, I was not who I used to be physically. Going gently was a continuing part of my path in order to stay well and, more importantly, to treat myself kindly.

Soon after those experiences with Jeff and the reduction of pain levels, I rose from bed one morning in an unfamiliar mood. As my feet hit the floor, my thoughts were of dread in going to work that day. Usually I loved being in my office, hearing the birds twitter as I looked out at trees and worked. It was not the case on this particular day. In fact, it was a long way off. I almost felt as if I hated my work.

While showering I realized it was not my work I hated. It was the pressure I had put on myself. As one project was coming to a close, I'd been jotting ideas down for the next. In that moment, I saw my heart was not into the new project at all. Its planning had come about from the suggestion of others in my working life, as something expected of me.

I had never followed the crowd, though, and had survived financially. My youth and distant past had once conditioned me to go into the corporate world of Monday to Friday. My heart had insisted otherwise. Being self-employed on the creative path was indeed a dream come true. It was also one I had courageously manifested for myself. There was much to be grateful for. As a solo parent, the only breadwinner in our little family, I was not just surviving financially anymore. I was living comfortably.

There was no need to start following the crowd now. Living life on my own terms was what I did best. It was the direction I needed to continue in. Work, particularly the new project, was feeling too much like work. I didn't want to work. I wanted to serve and create. There was a big difference. Yes, I had to generate and remain open to the flow of money. We all need it. I was enjoying the broader choices I now had than when existing in poverty. But if my heart was not into it, then it was wasted energy.

Removing the new project from future plans was liberating. There was no point putting my energy in its direction any longer. I couldn't do it with heart so I couldn't do it. The lessons of balance, given through being ill, had also called me back immediately. I had intended to take on too much for my wellbeing and enjoyment. The pressure was not healthy and demanded to be released.

It felt wonderful as yet another conscious choice toward feeling good was made. If it was not going to feel positive, it would have been created without authenticity. It would never have resonated peacefully with my values or existence.

The next choice I made was to give myself a day off to go wherever my heart led. Once out of work or solution-finding mode, inspiration flowed instantly. My heart was happy again. It had been heard and honored, so it spoke with renewed clarity. It was time to put my energy into fresh directions.

The unfolding speaking career was a fun change, particularly when doing my own events. I loved the joy the audience and I shared. As my message and intention were increasingly about getting offline and enjoying real-life connections, it made sense to place more focus in that direction. Smiley emoticons would never replace the delight of physical smiles and laughter the audience and I experienced at live events.

The message of kindness was also increasingly important. Every one of us needs more kindness from ourselves and one another. Our beloved planet and all her inhabitants desperately need more too. Shifting my own consciousness had demonstrated this was where true lasting transformation had to unfold. It would only be through a global shift in consciousness that kindness could flow unhindered. Supporting that shift was a direction calling me quietly but surely.

The heart continued to speak. It was calling me to serve again, in a balanced way this time. New directions were coming, even though their full vision was still being revealed. Other ideas surfaced, further confirming it was time to change route. Although service to others would be a part of my path, service to me was inherent for that to be possible.

There was no point in resistance. It was simply another call to growth.

60

One memorable day, while catching up with friends, I managed a fabulous swim out to the middle of a magnificent lake. It was surrounded by tea trees, which left an almost invisible film of soothing oil on the water. Both my body and skin felt softly nurtured by time in it. I loved the place and knew it well from another chapter in my past. It felt amazing to be swimming again. As my shoulders supported my arms through their cycles, my tender wrists handled the water's resistance with improved strength. My thoughts naturally floated to gratitude, for the experience of feeling free.

Once I'd swum far enough out that I could no longer hear conversations near the shore, I floated on my back, arms outstretched. With closed eyes, only my breathing could be heard. Shades of deep orange danced beyond my eyelids as the sun's rays warmed them. It was clear this lake would continue to play a role in my healing and rehabilitation.

It was heaven to be floating there at the center. I surrendered in peaceful trust to the rhythm of the lake's gentle sway. Reflecting on the previous four years, I considered who I was when entering them. I had thought that I was doing well. But back then, my standards of what "well" was were still ingrained in such low self-worth that "well" was not actually particularly great.

Now "doing well" was true to its meaning. I *was* doing well. Decisions were based not on fear, avoidance, or catering to the opinions of others. They were made solely on the loving guidance of my soul toward self-kindness, balance, and enjoyment. The space within both my heart and mind allowed for ease and much more gentleness and happiness.

Later that day, once home, I looked at the eyes in the mirror, ones that had known life experience, hardship, and heartbreaking pain. Yet more clearly, they revealed contentment, love, and a certainty of peace. I saw a secret happiness, one that revealed itself unhindered when the eyes broke into a smile.

A face once surrounded by long hair had faded into the past. The short hair, which had come about through the pain, now represented a lighter, freer spirit in every way. I no longer hid from who I was here to be. My smile represented a heart connected with self-love, shared with the confidence to be myself completely.

Any remnants of disease were now a gift rather than something to fight or resist. With another reduction successful, only half a weekly tablet remained. From the moment my focus had shifted to the divine intelligence within, it was clear a gradual reversal of disease was under way. Every step forward reminded me it was indeed a journey. Life was change. It was growth.

There would always be another lesson waiting. I could either view each one as a challenge or as another call to rise into my best self. By embracing the growth, enabling my resistance to dissolve and the learning to reveal itself more gently, I continued to find beauty amongst the so-called imperfection.

Rheumatoid arthritis had been one of my greatest teachers and despite appearances at times, one of the most loving. Just as I had developed a great love of de-cluttering my belongings, RA had helped me de-clutter things inside me emotionally and physically. Perhaps it would continue teaching me for some time to come or it would depart completely in the near future. Whatever would be was actually fine. My trust in its teachings was strong.

In its own way, RA had given me the best state of health and diet I'd ever known. As my perspective on wellness had changed, I felt remarkable. My body remained determined, insisting I treat both it and myself with ongoing, nurturing love. It was certainly a commitment I was willing to honor. More than anything, my journey through it had woken me to gratitude and conscious choice.

When things were at their absolute worst, when Elena was just a young toddler and I was petrified of every step I tried to take, one of my sisters went overseas on a work trip. She decided to take her daughter, who was about six at the time, with her. I remember thinking, *Imagine being that free.* Wrapping my head around the concept of independence, freedom, and traveling was too hard. It was a notion I could no longer grasp at all. It was also certainly not one that I could ever imagine for myself again.

Now I did feel free simply because I could walk up and down stairs unaided and I had the confidence to go to a market with Elena. The fact that I had been able to travel overseas with her and on my own still astounded me. I couldn't help but be grateful.

Guitar playing was still proving to be a challenge. My playing was disjointed and nowhere near what I knew once, but at least it was happening a tiny bit. There were occasions when grief for the old flow still surfaced. I allowed those feelings to be what they were. On other occasions, feeling better, I would try again.

One peaceful night while doing just that, I noticed the top knuckle of one of my fingers bent to hold the string, like in the old days. The middle knuckle of that finger was still rigid, but so had been the top one previously. Now it moved, just a couple of millimeters, but it was enough. The improvement was so subtle it was almost unnoticeable. Yet through that tiny action, I was given the gift of hope.

For the first time in years, I could genuinely visualize myself playing guitar loosely and happily again. It didn't matter that it was not in that very moment exactly. That would have been ridiculously wonderful, but I trusted in the journey now. In fact, I looked forward to what I would discover about myself through the ongoing rehabilitation of my wrists, hands, and fingers. There was no doubt it would bring joy on brand-new levels.

Improved wellness in all areas was something I had to look forward to. But the journey had taught me to not depend on it. Instead, by living as presently as I could, there were already moments of bliss to be found.

True peace did not depend on a result as much as a connection with my own divinity, with presence, and with love. I could never have once imagined it would actually be pain that would be the giver of those gifts to me. But indeed it was.

Peace through pain—that had always been one of the loving intentions of the lesson, to experience true peace in who I am.

61

My heart knew the next residence would be home. More and more I came to understand why I had not been ready before and why I was becoming more so now.

One thing I had never completely considered when first longing for the house on the hill was that I might actually share it with a partner. When those feelings for Jeff had burst my heart open initially, one of the very first fears that surfaced was of losing my independence by living together.

As time had since unfolded and layers of fear healed, I had opened up to the idea of living with my soul partner, whomever he might be. If I truly wanted to see the relationship reach its absolute potential of love, which I did, then there needed to be a continued willingness to surrender. The home that was waiting actually had to suit more than just me and Elena. It had to suit my partner, too. This realization gave me added patience and trust.

So many of my ideas about life had been completely shattered since becoming a mother and living through the intensity of pain I had. *Allowing* also felt much more natural than resisting. My connection and trust in God, in the big picture, and in the perfection of my universal journey was solid. With love and awe, my heart swelled often for how things had turned out.

In embracing the learning I had done through my feelings for Jeff, as well as the courage in sharing them, something had been brought out in me for which I was enormously grateful. I was much more connected with the woman I had become. As my body started shifting into a new cycle, through menopause, I felt even more grounded and empowered. It was safe to be me. It always had been but now I exercised that power. My connection with nature and its own cycles grew stronger, calling me home into myself until there was no separation from it at all.

Fears that had created walls of false self-protection for years were gone. My heart was courageous. It understood that love was not black and white. Nor was it clearly defined or linear, dictated by the beliefs of whatever culture we've been raised in. Only the heart knew best, not the opinions, belief systems, or social stigma that confronted us repeatedly on a daily basis.

Love was the air I breathed, the tears I cried, and the flower that opened. It was the frustration of trying to understand my lessons, the smile from a stranger, and the loved one who died.

With every new opinion formed, every old ideal released, or every conscious act of courage undertaken, my connection with the true language of my heart was increased. *Everything* I learned offered the opportunity to strip away man-made belief systems and reconnect to my soul and the big picture of my journey. And that is love.

Feeling that flow through my journey so far, my ability to surrender and allow was ever increasing. Life loved me. It had shown me so repeatedly. Every single one of my lessons was given from a place of love, with the intention to dissolve fear and bring me into my best self. All was well.

As a woman still in an earthly existence, I did continue to anticipate knowing my soul partner. It wasn't a romantic movie I was after. It was real life, with all our humanness revealed. I wanted to be conscious enough to create a mutual partnership with no goalposts we each had to meet to keep the other happy.

Through the bliss of surrender and acceptance that I had come to know, I would discover other parts of myself. I loved the idea of further self-discovery, even though I was aware it would stretch me. Resistance would surely surface as old fears and belief systems rose up and out. That was okay. It would be safe. The peaceful strength I had experienced through the vulnerability of honesty would accompany me through. I felt more ready than I ever had.

With my life no longer being aligned with the word *should* in other areas, I also intended to apply that to the relationship. Rather than having a fixed view of how things "should" be, I wanted to let myself be surprised. Through the acceptance of what is, each new revelation could then become a beautiful wonder. It was also my desire to support my partner in being his best self, as whoever he dreamed to be.

Returning sex to a sacred place was an intention, and this could be attained only through further acts of surrender. I was being called to view my sensuality entirely through the spiritual. That still allowed for the mischief and fun of tangling toes through laughter, but the call to fully experience surrender on every level was undeniable.

There was much to look forward to while still remaining as present as possible in the meantime. Happiness was being experienced on all sorts of new levels different from anything I'd known in my perception of it before. My heart heard its calling and would continue to trust in timing.

Life could surprise me, whenever it was ready—whenever *I* was ready.

62

Increasingly my friendships reflected the state of my mind. I was drawn only to positive people. It didn't mean we couldn't or didn't speak on topics of great depth. We did, but there was also space for lightness. I found myself prioritizing these friendships over others. I felt much more at home amongst happy, optimistic people. It was a direct reflection of my own brightness toward life again.

Shadows of pain no longer hindered me. Darkness was gone from my spirit. I was blossoming indeed, leaving gloom far behind. There would always be more growth, more lessons. No longer was there any conscious resistance to them, though. I was a strong woman, powerful and peaceful in her own essence. Whatever would be would be.

In allowing spirit to lead my work, too, unconventional opportunities continued floating in with ease. Sometimes they came from the previous years of hard work, from seeds already planted. At other times, they arrived through unexpected moments of synchronicity: being in the right place at the right time or falling into a conversation with a stranger. There was no need to strive. I only had to allow, which I did with open arms and a very open heart.

I had also just signed a movie deal for my first book. As having my life made into film was not actually something I craved, I had been in no hurry to sign in previous years when offers had come in. Having reached a place of surrendering and allowing, I now trusted that sharing my message further would not only benefit others, but my own soul's growth.

It was a matter of readiness and timing. Other random gifts also floated in easily. I was introduced to a holistic chef who prepared meals in people's homes. She was a lovely woman, around my age, who had chosen not to have children. Instead she gave her mothering energy to her work, nurturing me through loving intention as she cooked. Her wage was very reasonable and she required no commitment to a regular timetable. Instead, she was happy for me to call as needed. All I had to do was fill my fridge and pantry with foods I ate. Then she arrived and weaved her magic for a few hours. As a result, the fridge and freezer were full of divine meals inspired by creativity different from my own. Her help was the perfect occasional treat.

With my health improved, it was a joy to recognize that new thought patterns were now my natural way of thinking. It was okay to live gently. There was no achievement or success in busyness. My pace of life was healthy. There was no guilt in saying no.

With the growing call to be offline, while still accepting further growth in my career, it was time to employ a fabulous assistant. Views for additional team members further along also existed. The perfect person came along easily, a delightful woman with warmth and aligned professional skills. Work became enjoyable again, while still allowing space for fresh air, motherhood, real life relationships, movement, and ease.

I was a woman confident to be herself, dropping any expected formulas used in the world of entrepreneurs, artists, or self-employment. The only formula to follow was to courageously honor my heart's voice and enjoy life as fully as possible.

They say that the slowest-growing seeds bear the most fruit. It had certainly felt like that. For a long time it seemed like the seeds I had sown were not sprouting at all, but with faith, I continued to nurture them. Through surrender, God took over the role. Even when my fear and humanness lost hope, divine love was always still there caring for them, waiting for my readiness.

As I continued to grasp those ever-deepening lessons, seeds did begin blooming. Even the ease of the holistic chef coming into my life, something that was a far-fetched whimsical dream, reassured me I was not alone on this journey. Never had I been, not once. My prayers had always been heard. They always would be.

God was on my side. Life loved me.

63

It could have been easy to hope for a different ending to this tale. Once, I might have been hugely disappointed to not have the "ideal" ending. How would it look to others with an open finish? *What! She didn't get the man, or the house, or the complete remission of the disease?* Not yet, but I got *much* more. I was given freedom.

No longer was my life shaped by how it would be perceived by others. And no longer did I need to control the outcome. These two shifts were better than any physical detail arriving in my life before its right time.

To meet the expectations of how things "should" be, my story could have ended differently:

One morning I awoke with no pain at all in my body. My once-rigid fingers and tender hands felt loose, strong, and eager (despite certain muscles not having been at all active for almost five years). In my sexy silk nightgown I joyfully skipped on pain-free feet straight to my guitar.

I couldn't stop singing and playing. Music from heaven floated through me and out into the neighborhood. At the same moment, a handsome, broad-shouldered stranger was walking by, selling his organic fruit door-to-door. In a haze, a magic spell entranced him and he walked straight to my door.

I put my guitar aside, stood, and met him. (Of course, I looked absolutely ravishing in my silky gown, despite my hair still sticking up all over the place from the recent sleep.) Neither of us spoke a word. I just opened the door. He came in, putting his box of tropical fruit down before closing the door behind him. With his strong arms, he lifted me silently and carried me to the bedroom, which he naturally already knew the way to.

For days the world was forgotten, including how to care for my daughter, as we made slow, easy love behind closed curtains. We hardly

left the bed, eating only the grapes of love and feeding each other man-
goes from his tropical fruit box, kissing the juice from each other's chin.

When we did eventually float back into the world, we just happened
to walk past a real-estate window first. And there it was, our dream
castle on a hill. We bought it on the spot, without inspection, just know-
ing it was meant for us. And we lived happily ever after, with no bumps,
lessons, fears, or growth to ever worry about again.

Oh, and Elena was the flower girl at our wedding.

What an ending that could have been!

It is so easy to have preconceived ideas as to how something
should turn out. Yet the truth was the outcome of my journey felt
even better than the fantasy tale ever could have for me.

Having an ideal ending would have only been another pre-
conception of what perfection was. Instead, perfection was that
every moment itself is perfect. Every stage of my evolution was
absolutely right for that moment in time.

Health, romance, and home were all coming. My prayers had
been heard, without a doubt. The difference was that now they
were coming to a woman who was actually ready for the very best
of them all. The standards of my expectations had increased significantly through the journey.

There were no longer upper limits on what was possible. I
didn't have to settle for mediocre. It was real love I was expecting. Home could be heaven on earth, with a sense of heart and
stability like I'd never known previously. Health was appreciated
on new, sacred, and genuine levels for the miraculous gift it was.
Self-love and self-kindness were my new way of life, no longer just
ideals to aspire to.

Living without limits was being who God had always wanted
me to be. My needs would always be met. They always were, but
now I could hand it over, instead of trying to dictate just how
things should be.

It took searing pain to teach me the true beauty of perfection
and to extend my awe. There is magnificence in life, hidden daily,
waiting only for our vision to be clear enough to see it. We see
it best with our hearts. The only way to do that is to gradually
remove the haze of fear, conditioning, and preconceived ideas of

how our dreams *must* unfold. Allowing life to lead the way, knowing it has been the most loyal listener to our heart forever, is how we see that magnificence.

My dream was answered. More than anything it had been to know true happiness. I had also wanted to allow myself to do so free of guilt or shame. That gift was certainly given to me. Little did I know that through such a yearning, life would also teach me the power and joy of surrender, the strength in frailty, and the freedom of authenticity.

My journey would continue, but like the lotus flower that blooms through mud, I had finally learned to open myself up to the sunshine.

AFTERWORD

Upon the completion of this book, I felt like any mother who had just given birth: tender and a little emotional. Being called to bring this creation through and guiding its first steps has certainly been an honor. Knowing that I also have to now let it go, trusting it will take on a life of its own in the world, is yet another layer of surrender.

Despite considering myself a very private person, I have repeatedly been called to share my most vulnerable self while working through pain. It was certainly not a conscious desire to share my frailties so widely. The desire, instead, has been to honor my own heart and this is where it has led me.

While I was writing the last chapters, Elena was having a full and exciting mini-holiday down at her grandma's house with all her extended family. So I was free to celebrate the conclusion of this writing journey in my own way, having no idea at all there was this Afterword section to come.

I went to a local beach and watched the dusk settle in. It was a balmy summer night. The openness of the ocean was freeing, the sea breeze refreshing. I then had a magnificent massage. Once home, my body let go into a deep, restful sleep before I headed off the next morning, on the long drive to collect Elena.

After a couple of lovely days with Mum, my little darling girl and I hit the road home. There were many stories to share and the usual fun-filled conversations that unfold on our road trips. We spotted a café and decided to stop there for lunch. There was a

picnic table in a little grassy area between the café and the highway. Further afield were lush cane fields and mountains. The natural outlook was perfect for our short stop.

My meal was delicious. As Elena ate her own, I managed to
unscrew the lid off her drink with my hands instead of my teeth.
Any such achievements were always celebrated between us. We
carried on in ridiculous fun by raising our hands in the air and
cheering out loud. (An onlooker could never have imagined what
that cheer and laughter truly meant.)

Just as Elena returned to eating her lunch, the smile was wiped
from my face. A car was flying through the air, straight toward us.
It was as if it were in slow motion. As high as a bungalow, there it
was somersaulting through the air. As "Holy shit" came out of my
mouth, Elena looked up to witness it. The car then hit an electric-
ity pole, where it was bounced to the ground at full speed. From
there, it seemed to shift from slow motion into full rapid force.
With terrifying power, it rolled and rolled toward us.

The whole event was happening in a matter of seconds, not
minutes. *It's going to stop*, I thought. *It's going to stop?* Clearly, at the
pace it was coming at us, it was not. I scooped Elena up and ran,
probably for the first time in five years. A tree was a short distance
away. As I curled down hiding behind it, protecting Elena, I wondered if the tree was actually big enough to sustain the impact. I
realized it would not be, but there was nowhere else to go. We were
in God's hands.

The further sounds of crushing metal and an immediate eerie
silence told me the car had come to a stop. We were safe. We
were alive.

As we came out from behind the tree, somewhat stunned, a
man nearby rushed through the cloud of dust to the occupants of
the car. A woman rushed to the other side of it. Other people also
joined to help.

Knowing they were being attended to and that I had a little
girl to protect from what had just happened, I did the best thing
I could. I jumped straight onto the phone to emergency services,
while still cuddling Elena. She was upset because shrapnel and
mud from the car's slide had landed on her lunch, ruining it. The

top of her foot also had a small splinter land in it. Thank goodness her mind did not fully grasp the extent of what we'd just seen. Other people came over and chatted with her, too.

While on the phone I had to walk to the crashed car, which had stopped only about five meters from our picnic table. It was necessary for me to tell the operator what I could see. So while Elena waited with the other folks briefly, I went closer. Despite having worked with death for years, it felt strange to see people so close to it again. The cold, crushing metal felt like such an unreal contrast to the soft, floppy bodies inside.

An elderly woman was in the passenger's side, alive but clearly in shock, with bleeding hands and unable to move her legs properly. The driver, an elderly man, looked dead; his head flopped forward at a strange angle. I couldn't see his breath from the other side of the car, but the angel who first ran to them said he was still breathing. That man helping was meant to be there, without a doubt. The way he handled the patients made it clear he knew this line of work.

Several minutes were spent on the phone, even after returning to hold Elena some more. Finally, once that was done, we just sat and held each other. I nuzzled her little head into me and held her to my heart like never before. Once the emergency services arrived, I was free to go. They had my phone number and would call if they needed any further information.

As we headed off, Elena asked lots of questions to process things at her own level. "Who was inside the car?" Two old people, I told her. "Are they hurt?" So I explained about the woman's bleeding hand. "How do they fix it?" A discussion about medical stitches followed. "Has the man hurt his hand, too?" No, I said, he'd hurt his head. "Is the man going to die?" I didn't know, I told her, but thought he might. (I found out the next day that he had died on the way to hospital. Bless his soul.) "Who's going to pick up all their things for them?" (Their belongings had been strewn across the park from the impact.) The policeman would do that, I said. "How will the woman get home from hospital if she doesn't have a car and he dies?" On and on the questions went. Hearing it from her perspective, and also noticing the empathy that naturally flowed from her, was precious.

It was interesting she had been introduced to death so early on in life. She still asked questions about my dad being gone and was quite matter-of-fact about it occurring to people, animals, and plants. Her fascination was pure, innocent, and honest. Death had shaped my own life immensely, especially caring for dying people. Now it seemed as though it was to be a part of her lineage for me to pass on my knowledge of the subject, as a natural part of our conversations. I was grateful for the openness on such an essential topic.

We drove on, but I realized I also needed a hug. There was too much thick energy hanging around me that I didn't want to take home. I needed to wash it off. So I called a friend, who offered her listening ear. About an hour further into the trip, we met her at the tea-tree lake. While she played with Elena and did her own healing with her, I was able to swim.

I felt the strongest I had in years as I gently pushed my body further and further out. There was no denying I was in a strange space myself, including feeling more alive than ever. Adrenaline from coming so close to even my own death possibly shaped this. Still, I couldn't shake the woman's shocked face and the man's loose body from my vision. I knew I would find my own way to process it, including the prayers I would say for her and for his soul. But swimming was the first step to shifting things. The lake drew the energy from me, lifting it out of the water and away.

By the time we arrived home in the late afternoon, we both felt okay, considering. We did drawings of the event and it was clear Elena was going to be fine, not having seen inside the car. She could be affected only by the vision of the crumpled metal and our need to hide. There was no denying I felt even closer to her afterward than I ever had. This reminder of how quickly life can change reinforced my resolution to continue living my best life.

Weeks have rolled into months and we keep moving forward. The truth of readiness and timing has since been revealed with unstoppable momentum.

My body continues to grow stronger at its own pace. On one particularly glorious morning another level of confidence was returned, when I rode a bicycle. It was exhilarating to realize my wrists and hands were strong enough to control it. My knee joints could pedal without pain. Riding along a bike path with the ocean by my side, I celebrated freedom. Soon after, I purchased my own bike and now ride regularly. I love the view of life from this pace.

With Elena a little older and not so inclined to climb all over me when I stretch, a gradual home practice of yoga has returned. Regular massages have also become a part of my routine, rather than just something I did when reaching exhaustion. The ongoing maintenance has made the world of difference to my wellbeing.

On a sunny afternoon life crossed my path with a new friend. Conversation and humor flowed between us as if we'd known each other forever. Within a few hours of meeting him, I realized I hadn't needed a 25-year friendship. I had just needed to reach a place in myself where it always felt safe to be me. A beautiful friendship began that afternoon, taking us by wonderful surprise. There is a lot of smiling going on for us both.

Another forward step has been to contract another team member, a remarkable man with international experience perfect for my new directions. Other professionals also assist us all. It feels incredible to experience the support of a growing, enthusiastic team.

Increasingly, our little villa has proven to be absolutely perfect for our current lifestyle. The yearning for a different home has subsided as I am at home in my heart. A wave of gratitude hits every time I return to our sweet little place from further travels. Simply having *a* home, a base to return to, is abundance in itself. Being low-maintenance care is an added bonus. We just shut the door and go.

I am enjoying the best of both worlds—the freedom of travel and the comfort of a lovely home. It is ideal. My heart definitely wants to continue living as simply as possible, and, in this moment, my needs have been met. The practice of surrender continues to be a gift of freedom. It allows the future to flow however life sees as best for me.

After a fabulous three-week detox experience in an Ayurvedic hospital in India, I said goodbye to the last of the pharmaceutical medications. Symptoms of RA decreased noticeably and my strength improved. I view any remaining symptoms as loving reminders to always go gently, to make the right choices supporting my wellbeing and joy. Subtle improvements continue, so their role grows more redundant by the day. Going gently is now my way of life.

It is time to step away from the computer some more and reconnect with other expressions of creativity, including guitar playing and songwriting. My fingers are longing to reawaken. This is my new commitment. Despite the challenge ahead, I feel positive.

Time is a gift. Regardless of what age we may or may not live to, it still flies by quickly. To recognize and respect just how fragile life really is helps us to see how precious its offering is. This is all the more reason to be authentic, courageous, and grateful.

We are here to live our very best life. We will be pulled out of our comfort zones. There will be resistance, fear, anger, and sadness. But if we dare to allow it, there will be laughter and magnificence, too.

It is okay to show our frailty and to share our honesty. In fact, it is fabulous to do so. Life loves us and wants to bestow the largest dose of happiness possible upon us.

We just need the courage to allow it.

ACKNOWLEDGMENTS

My heartfelt thanks to all who have shared this journey with me, and through my other books, songs, live events, mailing list, blog, and social media. Your presence is felt, loved, and gratefully enjoyed. Thank you to those in my inner circle for your love and sustenance. And thank you to all with the courage to honor your heart's voice. You are making the world a better place for us all, including me. I thank you and send you love.

ABOUT THE AUTHOR

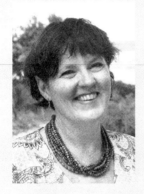

Bronnie Ware is the author of the international bestselling memoir *The Top Five Regrets of the Dying: A Life Transformed by the Dearly Departing*, published in 29 languages worldwide. In December 2015, Enigma Films optioned the rights to make *The Top Five Regrets of the Dying* into a full-length feature film. Her second book, *Your Year for Change: 52 Reflections for Regret-Free Living*, has also been translated into numerous languages.

Bronnie's calling is to lead by courageous example. Her grounded attitude and sense of humour are often commented on at live events. Having sat by bedsides of the terminally ill for several years, Bronnie knows the pain of dying with regret. She also understands the value of humour and authenticity. Consequently, she honours these remarkably by bravely exercising her power of choice with consciousness and courage on a daily basis.

As well as being an author, Bronnie is an inspirational speaker and a songwriter. Some of her favorite things are to combine her talents into fun-filled stage presentations, as well as getting people off their computers and back to real-life conversations and experiences.

Her favourite role is as a mother. Her favourite teacher is nature.

Bronnie lives in New South Wales, Australia.

www.bronnieware.com

Hay House Titles of Related Interest

YOU CAN HEAL YOUR LIFE, the movie,
starring Louise Hay & Friends
(available as a 1-DVD program and an expanded 2-DVD set)
Watch the trailer at: www.LouiseHayMovie.com

THE SHIFT, the movie,
starring Dr. Wayne W. Dyer
(available as a 1-DVD program and an expanded 2-DVD set)
Watch the trailer at: www.DyerMovie.com

All of the above are available at www.hayhouse.co.uk

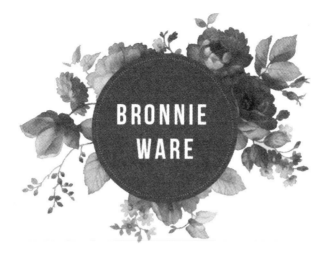

BRONNIE WARE

LIVE TRUE TO YOUR HEART'S OWN SONG

I was recently asked by an audience member if I was a naturally confident person or whether I have been more motivated by courage. Through this journey in *Bloom,* it may seem like I was both.

But it hasn't always been this way.

**JOIN ME AS I TALK ABOUT COURAGE AND HOW
I USE IT TO SUPPORT MY ONGOING JOURNEY:**

www.bronnieware.com/bloom

My first memoir, *The Top Five Regrets of the Dying,* shares the start of the journey into my true self. While sitting beside the beds of dying people, my own life was gradually transformed through the regrets they shared with me.

www.bronnieware.com/regrets-of-the-dying

To discover more of Bronnie's work, and for information on upcoming events and workshops, visit: www.bronnieware.com

BRONNIE'S SONGS ARE AVAILABLE FROM DIGITAL STORES WORLDWIDE.

 facebook.com/bronnieware instagram.com/bronnie.ware

NOTES

NOTES

NOTES

NOTES

HAY HOUSE

Look within

Join the conversation about latest products,
events, exclusive offers and more.

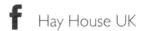 Hay House UK

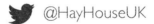 @HayHouseUK

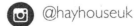 @hayhouseuk

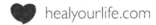 healyourlife.com

We'd love to hear from you!